The Simple Heart Cure Diet and Meal Plan

The Simple Heart Cure Diet and Meal Plan

28 Days of Healthy Meals and Over 100 Delicious and Easy Recipes

Chauncey Crandall, M.D.

with

Charlotte Libov

Humanix Books

THE SIMPLE HEART CURE DIET AND MEAL PLAN

Humanix Books, P.O. Box 20989, West Palm Beach, FL 33416, USA

www.humanixbooks.com | info@humanixbooks.com

Humanix Books is a division of Humanix Publishing, LLC. Its trademark, consisting of the words "Humanix Books," is registered in the Patent and Trademark Office and in other countries.

Disclaimer: The information presented in this book is not specific medical advice for any individual and should not substitute medical advice from a health professional. If you have (or think you may have) a medical problem, speak to your doctor or a health professional immediately about your risk and possible treatments. Do not engage in any care or treatment without consulting a medical professional.

ISBN: 9-781-63006-123-4 (Hardcover)
ISBN: 9-781-63006-124-1 (E-book)

Printed in the United States of America

10 9 8 7 6 5 4 3 2 1

To my wife, Deborah; my sons, Christian and Chad; and "my tribe," the patients the Lord has entrusted to my care. Also, to the many great physicians and professors who taught me about the art and science of medicine and caring for those in need.

CONTENTS

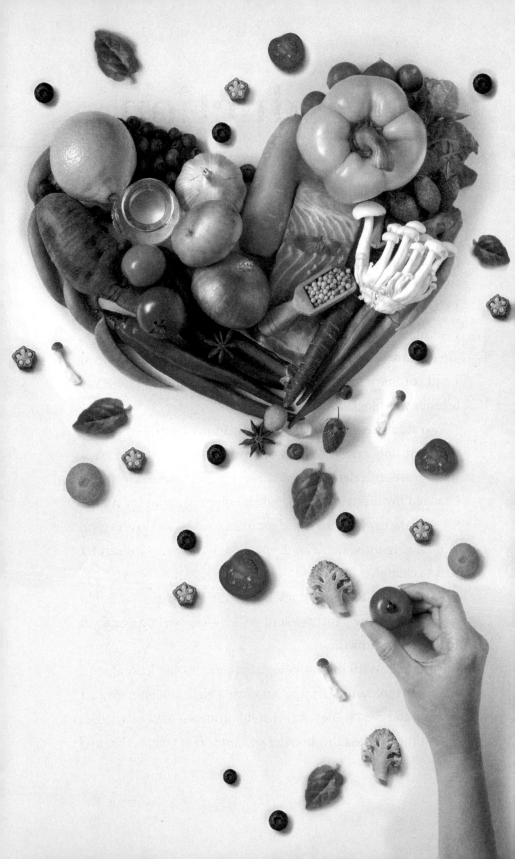

Introduction

Twenty years ago, I found myself in a crisis on the brink of a heart attack.

A few days earlier, I'd felt a pain in my left shoulder, which I assumed was a pulled muscle. But, after ignoring it, the pain continued to build up in intensity and did not decrease. Now, after an emergency trip to the hospital, here I was. I soon learned I had coronary heart disease, and the blood flow to one of my arteries was blocked.

Two stents restored the blood flow to my heart, but I knew they were only a possible short-term fix. I knew heart disease is a progressive and relentless disease process and, unless I drastically changed my lifestyle, there would be more issues in my future.

For years, my wife had urged me to eat healthy and lose weight, and I had ignored her. But, deep down, I knew she was right. I had to change.

So I decided to pour all my knowledge and experience into a plan to help my patients—and myself—lose weight and stick to a heart-healthy diet.

It worked. With my cardiologist practice as my laboratory, I have seen thousands of my patients lose weight and reverse heart disease, and even I—despite my stubbornness—have succeeded.

And the result is this book, *The Simple Heart Cure Diet and Meal Plan.*

Why the Simple Heart Cure Diet Works

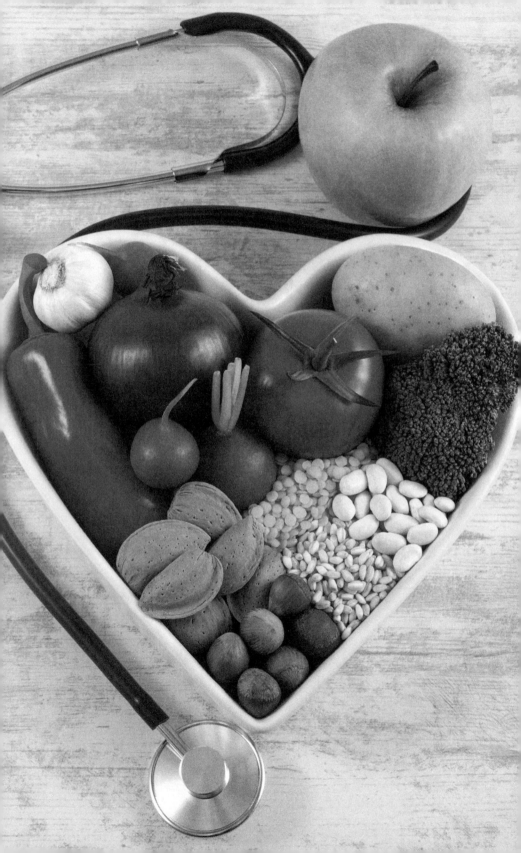

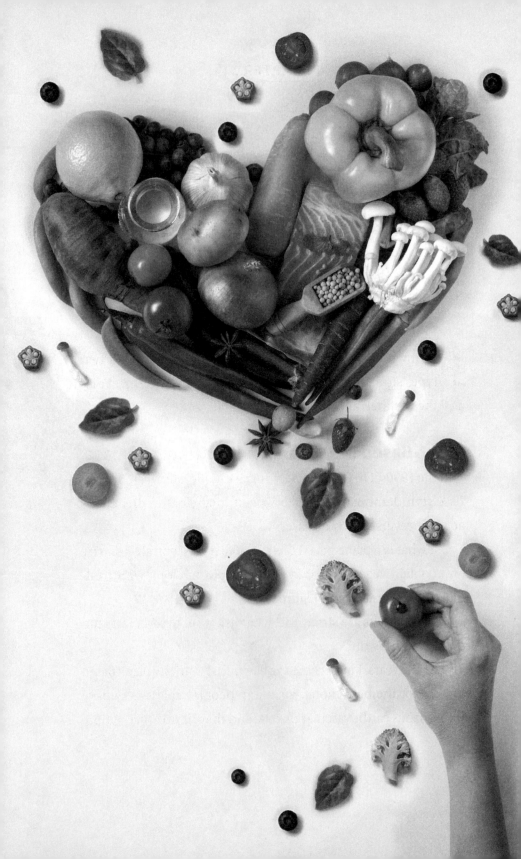

CHAPTER 1

Let's Get Started!

For my lifetime diet plan, I reviewed many diets, and two types stood out: the plant-based heart disease reversal diet and the Mediterranean diet.

Plant-Based Diets Can Reverse Heart Disease

In the 1990s, Dr. Dean Ornish and, a decade later, Dr. Caldwell Esselstyn demonstrated that a strict, plant-based diet could actually reverse heart disease.

Just what is a plant-based diet? It's a diet concentrated on raw and cooked vegetables of every description, along with fresh fruit, whole grains, and legumes (beans).

But these diets are strict, and what use is such a diet if it's too difficult to stay on?

Over the years, I have come to believe that a strictly plant-based diet is not the best choice for many people, unless they have very serious cardiovascular disease and there is no other option.

The Mediterranean Diet Is More Satisfying

On the other hand, the Mediterranean diet is one of the most studied and highly ranked diets in the world. It also contains foods in diets followed naturally by people living in the "Blue Zones," where an unusually high number of people who reach the age of 100 reside.

The problem is that the Mediterranean diet is more lenient than the plant-based heart reversal diets, so while it's easier to stick to, many people find it difficult to lose weight with it.

The Solution? The Simple Heart Cure Diet

So this was my challenge: to create a diet that would take some aspects of plant-based eating and combine it with aspects of the Mediterranean diet, which, while tasty and satisfying, does not necessarily achieve weight loss. So I took aspects of both to create a diet that is not only satisfying and delicious but also heart healthy.

Goals of the Simple Heart Cure Diet

The Simple Heart Cure Diet also helps reverse and prevent heart disease by reducing the following major heart disease risk factors:

- **high cholesterol**
- **high blood pressure**
- **diabetes and pre-diabetes**
- **obesity**

GOAL 1. Tackle High Cholesterol

If you have even mildly elevated cholesterol, you are likely concerned about your doctor putting you on statin drugs, which lower cholesterol but also carry potential side effects.

For my patients without underlying heart disease, I recommend a total cholesterol count of under 170–200 mg/dl. People with coronary heart disease need to keep their total cholesterol reading below 150.

Getting to your goal weight, which for most people is the weight they were in high school, will result in lowering your cholesterol.

GOAL 2. Lower High Blood Pressure

Because my diet is rich in fruits and vegetables as well as fiber, it naturally lowers high blood pressure.

GOAL 3. Prevent or Reverse Diabetes

About 29 million Americans, or 9% of the population, have the metabolic disorder known as diabetes, yet millions of them are unaware of it.

In addition, millions of additional Americans also have insulin resistance, which is also referred to as "prediabetes." This is sometimes also called "borderline" or "mild" diabetes, but don't be fooled. People in this category almost invariably go on to develop full-blown diabetes and heart disease. So if you're told you are insulin resistant, or have pre-diabetes, you have to treat the diagnosis just as seriously as if you had full-blown diabetes.

Losing weight on my diet will help you control your diabetes as well as prevent and even reverse it.

DR. CRANDALL'S MOTIVATIONAL TIP
Love Is the Greatest Motivator

Because I'm a cardiologist, my new patients often expect me to lecture them on the consequences that will befall them if they don't lose weight. But fear of death can only motivate you for a little while. In the end, it's what you truly love that determines whether or not you will take the steps to successfully lose weight. That is why love is the most powerful motivator in the world.

Do you love eating and drinking more than your family? More than what you might yet accomplish in your life? Have you given up, or do you want to live?

If you start eating as I've recommended, you'll feel so much better that you'll rediscover the joys in life. Eat right in order to live a life that's truly worth living—that's my Simple Heart Cure Diet Plan.

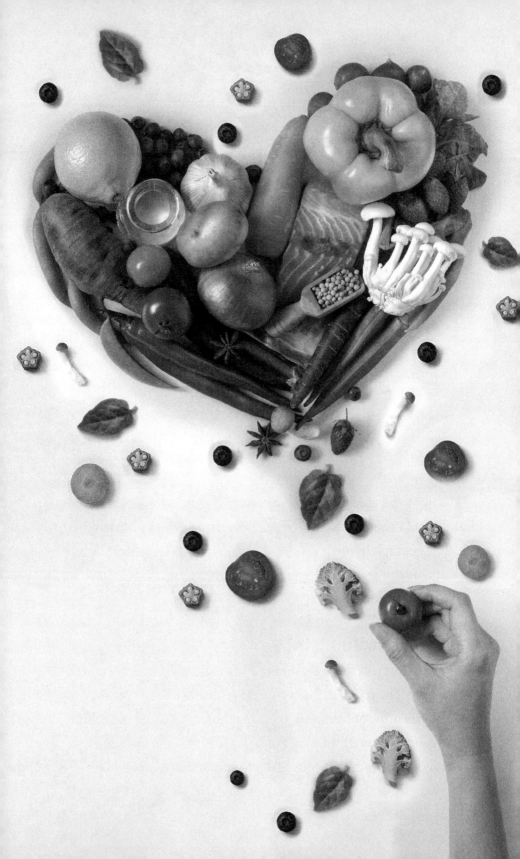

CHAPTER 2

The Principles of the Simple Heart Cure Diet

I'd like to be able to tell you that my diet contains some secret formula that no one has ever thought of before, bringing about a complete revolution in nutritional thinking. But, like most true things, my diet's wisdom is based on ideas that have been understood for ages.

You Have to Jump In!

My patients often ask me how they can implement such a diet gradually. The truth is, you can't. You must challenge yourself head-on. Throw out all the junk in your house, go shopping with a completely altered shopping list, and learn how to cook tasty, healthy meals from the foods I'll be recommending in this book.

Principle 1. Fill Up on Fruits and Vegetables

Much of it is as simple as what your mother told you: eat your fruits and vegetables.

Unlike grains and meat, fruits and vegetables send a clear signal to your brain that you are full, and it's time to stop eating.

Principle 2. Eat Protein Every Day

The major difference between my diet and a total plant-based diet involves animal protein. While it's possible to get protein from nonanimal sources, there is a real role for animal-based proteins in any diet. After all, human beings have been fishing and hunting wild game for eons. Today we have to be more cautious about the meats we eat because the way we get our food has changed so much.

Red meat should be avoided except on special occasions, and even poultry should be consumed in small portions. Because red meats should be an infrequent part of your diet, try to restrict your red meat to wild game such as bison and venison.

I recommend that most of your animal-based proteins come from fish. Fatty fish are rich in omega-3 oils; leaner fish are nutrient-rich without being high in calories.

Principle 3. Fill Up on Fiber

When it comes to eating a heart-healthy diet, fiber is a key way to reduce cholesterol and stay full longer, which reduces overeating.

There are two kinds of fiber: insoluble and soluble. Both types are important.

Insoluble fiber is indigestible fiber, the kind found in foods such as wheat bran, vegetables, and whole grains.

Soluble fiber attracts water and turns to gel, which slows digestion and can help you feel full longer. Soluble fiber is found in foods such as oat bran, barley, nuts, seeds, beans, lentils, and peas.

Principle 4. Chose the Right Fats

You can add small amounts of olive oil to your salads, with vinegar, for instance. People have been thriving for millennia on olive oil. It has tremendous antioxidant and healing properties.

When you are "dressing" a salad, remember to keep it skimpy. Use the oil sparingly in a vinaigrette dressing, and put your portion to the side where you can just dip your fork into it as needed.

The Simple Heart Cure Diet Plan in Action

Here is an example of my typical day following the Simple Heart Cure Diet. I eat like this every day, especially during the work week. On the weekend, my wife and I allow ourselves a little variety to keep the diet from feeling like a burden. That's OK as long as you go right back to the plan and stay with it.

In sum, keep it simple, keep it light, and keep it fresh. Find healthy foods you enjoy, and explore the whole world of seasonings that can make healthy meals into real taste treats.

- **6 a.m.** I kick-start my metabolism with a glass of water with lemon, then I go for an hour-long walk to get my blood flowing. Fresh air and gentle, moderate exercise help get the day started.
- **7 a.m.** When I come home, I have a breakfast of two egg whites and one egg yolk, sliced cucumber, sliced tomatoes, steamed spinach, one piece of whole grain toast with a little orange marmalade, and a cup of coffee. Whole grains are digested more slowly and evenly when they are combined with protein. Eggs even out the insulin production, and keep me feeling satisfied and energetic much longer.

  Not so long ago, I was eating only oatmeal and fruit in the morning; however, I ran out of energy at about 10 o'clock each morning. Even whole grain starches cause a pronounced rise in the secretion of insulin, which eventually leads to a sudden drop in blood sugar.
- **12 p.m.** For lunch, I have a salad with a strip of chicken or fish. I use very little dressing and always place it on the side. Once again, the protein helps the meal carry me through the afternoon. For variety, I'll make myself a sandwich of a small slice of hard cheese, avocado, and sliced turkey on whole wheat or other "whole" grain bread. Make sure the bread is whole grain, not "multigrain" or another type that has added sugar. No matter which grain you choose, the important term is *whole*, which means the entire kernel is used.

- **2:30 p.m.** A small handful of raw walnuts or almonds helps me get through a hungry spell in the mid-afternoon. I always have some nearby, just in case. If I get really hungry, I'll complement the nuts with an apple.
- **6 p.m.** For dinner, I have fish, steamed vegetables, and a bowl of fruit for dessert.

   Occasionally, I'll have a piece of dark chocolate as a healthy indulgence.

DR. CRANDALL'S MOTIVATIONAL TIP

Not Just a Heart Diet

I often tell my patients, "Save Your Heart, Save Your Life." You are entitled to victory!

This is because my diet isn't just a diet that will save your heart—by following it, you can save your life by steeply reducing your risk of developing the four major killer diseases:

- heart disease
- stroke
- cancer
- diabetes

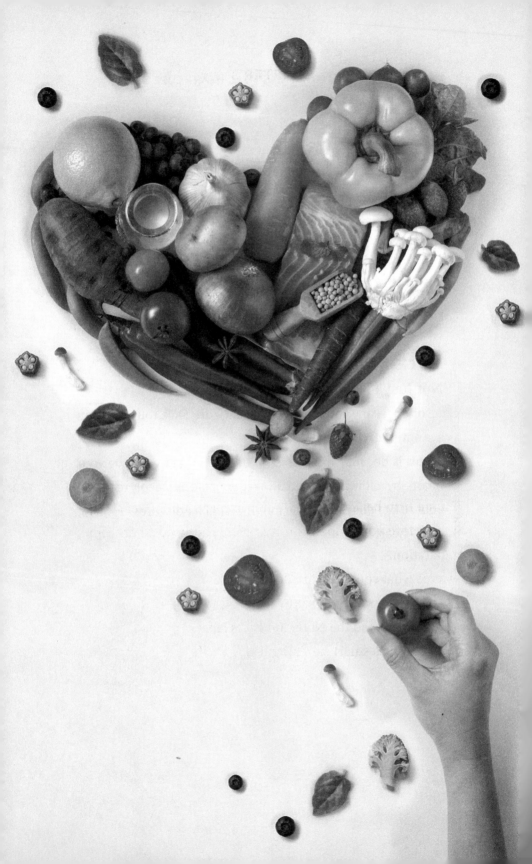

CHAPTER 3

How to Prepare for the Simple Heart Cure Diet

I am a firm believer in the motto Preparation Is Everything, so before you embark on this diet, you need to do some preparation.

Here's what you'll need to do:

1. Get rid of your unhealthy food.
2. Learn to read the Nutrition Facts label.
3. Compile a smart shopping list.

1. Get Rid of Unhealthy Food

Take action! Throw out or donate all your fat-laden, processed foods—you're not going to need them anymore. Clear it all out to make room for heart-healthy food! Toss out anything packaged, processed, or filled with chemicals. This includes chemically laden, low-fat foods. Do this to the food in your freezer and on your pantry or kitchen shelves. Don't worry about being wasteful—it's much better to clear this food out of your house for life.

2. Learn to Read the Nutrition Facts Label

In 1990, a law was enacted that resulted in the Nutrition Facts label you generally see on all packaged foods. This has made eating healthy far easier to do. Get to know the Nutrition Facts label; it provides you with a wealth of knowledge. Here's how to decipher it:

Serving size—This information shows how many servings the package contains. Too often, we assume that a single package of food is one serving, but if you read the label, you may find out that it contains two or more. So if you intend to eat the entire package, you may learn you're actually going to be consuming more calories, fat, and/or sugar than you had intended.

Calories—Calories provide a measure of how much energy each serving of food provides. The government uses 2,000 calories a day as a general yardstick, but the number varies depending on your age, gender, height, weight, and level of daily activity. My diet doesn't require you to count calories, because I advise you to eat as much whole food as possible, but if you're adding packaged foods, the calorie counts can guide you—or steer you away from them. In addition, each nutrient is marked with the percentage that it contributes to a daily diet of 2,000 calories. This is known as the "Percent Daily Value," and, for reference, 5% or less is considered low, and 20% or more is considered high.

Nutrients—A nutrient is a substance that provides nourishment essential for growth and maintenance of life. The nutrients spelled out on the nutritional label include total fat (and how much of that is saturated and trans fat), cholesterol, sodium, and total carbohydrates. The breakdown of these values for total carbohydrates must also be stipulated: dietary fiber and total sugars, including the percentage of added sugar. The amount of protein is also noted as well as these important vitamins:

- vitamin D
- calcium
- iron
- potassium

When it comes to nutrients, the key is to eat more of the ones you want and less of the ones you don't want.

Ingredients to Get Less Of: Saturated Fat, Sodium, and Added Sugars

Saturated fat, trans fat, sodium (salt), and added sugars are the ones you don't want; they are associated with obesity and chronic illnesses such as high blood pressure and diabetes, and, unfortunately, Americans tend to eat more of them. Added sugars tend to raise calorie counts as well as being generally unhealthy.

Fats: "Good Fats" vs. "Bad Fats"

The belief that all dietary fat is bad is off base; your body does need some fat to function. But it all depends on the type of fats; there are good fats and bad fats.

Saturated fat is found in higher proportions in animal products and is usually solid at room temperature. The Dietary Guidelines for Americans recommend consuming less than 10% of calories from saturated fats.

Trans fat is also unhealthy. These are fats formed artificially during food processing and are found in partially hydrogenated oils, which are used in a variety of foods, such as baked goods, coffee creamer, ready-to-use frostings, snack foods, and stick margarine.

As of 2018, most uses of partially hydrogenated oils—the major source of artificial trans fats in the U.S. food supply—have been phased out. Trans fat is also present at very low levels in refined vegetable oils.

For good health, the majority of the fats you eat should be monounsaturated or polyunsaturated. Eat foods containing monounsaturated fats and/or polyunsaturated fats instead of foods that contain saturated fats and/or trans fats.

Sugars: Total Sugars vs. Added Sugars

When the Nutrition Facts label was last revised in 2016, I was happy to see that an "added sugars" category had been included. Added sugars are sweeteners added to foods or beverages during processing, but they do not include naturally occurring sugars such as those in milk and fruits. The FDA recommends that people consume no more than 10% of their total daily calories from added sugar. The new labeling included those figures as well.

This label information is especially needed because discerning the actual amount of sugar in processed foods is quite difficult because sweeteners go by so many names. Among them: agave, brown rice syrup, corn sweetener, corn syrup, dextrin, dextrose, glucose, fructose, honey, invert sugar, lactose, maltodextrin, maltose, mannitol, molasses, natural sweeteners, polydextrose, sucrose, syrup, turbinado sugar, and xylitol.

And, although it's often obvious that some foods are sugar-laden, such as sweet desserts, sugared sodas, and cereals, some foods contain sugar even though you don't expect them to, such as salad dressings, barbecue sauces, and ketchups. Even some brands of toothpaste may contain sugar. I refer to these types of foods as containing "hidden" sugar, so reading the nutrition labels will enable you to ferret them out.

Nutrients to Get More Of: Dietary Fiber, Vitamin D, Calcium, Iron, and Potassium

Dietary fiber, vitamin D, calcium, iron and potassium are nutrients on the label that Americans generally do not get the recommended amount of and should look to get more of.

Eating a diet high in dietary fiber can increase the frequency of bowel movements, lower blood glucose and cholesterol levels, and reduce calorie intake. Diets higher in vitamin D, calcium, iron, and potassium can reduce the risk of developing osteoporosis, anemia, and high blood pressure.

3. Compile a Smart Shopping List

As any smart dieter will tell you, there are two things you should never do if you are serious about eating healthier—the first is to go food shopping when you're hungry, and the second is to go without a list and just wander the store.

Supermarkets today are laid out in a certain way, and too often there are landmines—areas where even the most stalwart dieter can run afoul because of foods that tempt you to indulge—like the displays of candy at the cash register, where you are going to have to wait a bit, for instance.

For those who find the supermarket too much of a temptation, you can avoid it altogether, thanks to services such as Instacart, Amazon Prime, and Walmart, to name a few, but most of us still like to do our shopping in person.

Whichever way you do your grocery shopping, you can use the information in the next chapter to stock up with the items you'll need, both to create your own recipes or use the ones in this book.

DR. CRANDALL'S MOTIVATIONAL TIP
Stick to Your List!

Take the time to organize your shopping list to mirror how you will walk through the supermarket. You'll get out of the store much faster, and with all the healthy foods you need (and want) and less chance of picking up an unhealthy impulse item.

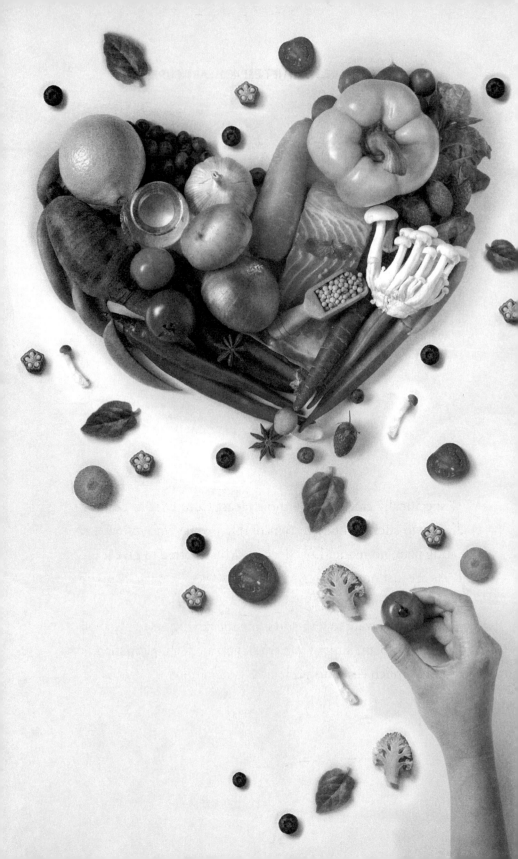

CHAPTER 4

How to Stick to the Simple Heart Cure Diet

I specifically crafted the Simple Heart Cure Diet to make it easy to stick to, but I recognize that people who follow any eating plan, no matter how good, will be tempted to give it up. Diets are just not easy to stick to; if they were, we would all be walking around slim as reeds.

That's why I want to give you some special secrets to help you stick to this plan. Simply put, when you are feeling satisfied, it becomes much easier to push away temptations.

Snack on Protein!

Hunger is a major reason people don't stick to their diets. Foods high in protein are good snacking choices because they help you feel fuller longer. Protein takes longer to digest than carbohydrates, so you'll feel satisfied, and the fuller you are, the less likely you are to reach for other snacks.

Every cell in our body uses protein for basic functioning. Protein produces the hormones that keep our organs and immune systems functioning. Protein also regulates our sleep and digestive symptoms. It repairs our muscles and connective tissues.

So, if you get hungry between meals, this feeling may be due to your body calling out its need for protein. One caveat, though: you must be careful about the foods you choose because some high-protein food may also be high in saturated fat, such as meat or full-fat cheese.

Here are ten good-for-you, high-protein snacks:

Hard-Boiled Eggs

Eggs are a high-protein snack. Boil a half dozen and keep them in the refrigerator for easy snacking. Eggs no longer have been found to raise cholesterol as much as once believed, but moderation is still the key, so limit yourself to one egg daily.

Nuts

Nuts are protein powerhouses that also contain fiber and heart-healthy oils. But they are also calorie-dense, so parcel them out in one-ounce serving packets. If you're looking for the lowest-calorie nut, that would be almonds, at 129 calories versus 172 for mixed nuts. Whichever nuts you choose, make sure they are unsalted.

Greek Yogurt

With twice the protein of regular yogurt, there is no reason not to choose Greek yogurt for snacking. But because flavored yogurts can be high in sugar, choose plain Greek yogurt, and mix in fresh fruits or berries.

Cottage Cheese

Choose low-fat or nonfat cottage cheese that you can enjoy with either diced fruits or raw vegetables. A half cup offers 14 grams of protein with 100 calories per serving.

Sliced Turkey

While my Simple Heart Cure Diet is largely plant based, there is leeway, especially when it comes to protein. Salmon (or other cold-water fish) is your best choice, but, when it comes to a portable snack, nothing beats sliced turkey. Three ounces of turkey is low in both fat and calories. Home-roasted turkey is best, but if you are buying it packaged, beware of added sodium or sugar.

Edamame

Half a cup of edamame, or fresh soybeans, provides 8 grams of protein for a 100-calorie snack. For added flavor, you can sprinkle lightly with reduced-sodium soy sauce.

Pumpkin Seeds

Like nuts, pumpkin seeds are easy to take along, and are also very rich in minerals, including potassium, manganese, and, especially, iron. Just take heed; they are also high in calories, so eat small amounts, such as about 1.5 ounces or ¼ cup.

Lentils

Like members of the bean group, lentils are packed with protein as well as fiber and lots of other nutrients, including a host of vitamins, minerals, amino acids, and more. They are also relatively quick to prepare, and, because they soak up the flavors of what they're cooked with, they are versatile and delicious. A cup of cooked lentils offers 18 grams of protein, but only 1 gram of fat.

Tofu

Tofu gets its nutritional punch because it's made from soy. Because it absorbs flavors so well, it can be prepared in a variety of ways as well, so you can use it for a meal and enjoy the leftovers as snacks.

Hummus

Hummus makes a tasty snack, especially when served with some celery or carrot sticks.

Did You Fall Off the Wagon? Get Back on It!

Sticking to your diet is the goal, but no one is perfect. We all mess up now and then! The main goal is to get back on your diet; remember, losing weight—and keeping it off—is a marathon, not a sprint!

Healthy Habits to Help Lose Weight—and Keep It Off

Think like a thin person. What is it about some people who never seem to struggle with their weight, yet remain slender no matter what they eat? No doubt you know some. What's their secret? Do they think differently than the rest of us do? The answer is yes!

People who don't struggle with food or weight use their natural signals of hunger and fullness to guide their eating. They don't need to think about food all the time because they trust their bodies to let them know when and how much to eat.

But what if you're not born this way? Here are some strategies that thin people naturally follow, and you can follow them as well.

Start the day with breakfast. "Don't skip breakfast." That's the finding of 78% of the participants enrolled in the National Weight Loss Registry, which is the largest ongoing research study of 10,000 people, who have not only lost weight but kept it off.

Build in exercise throughout the day. I'll get into my fitness plan later, but for now, keep in mind that, even though it was once thought you should exercise in one period, research now shows you can spread it throughout the day, and, by doing this, you can help reinforce your healthy eating habit!

Click off the TV and shut down the screens. We know a lot of people gained weight during the COVID-19 pandemic. We also know the pandemic ushered in the practice of binge-watching, where people watch an entire season of a show downloaded from a streaming network; they could be watched in one long marathon seating. Coincidence? I think not!

Instagram, Facebook, TikTok, and the like can also be time-sinks. They take your attention off of what you are eating, too. Binge-watching can lead to binge-eating!

Become a calorie counter—even unconsciously. Counting calories isn't a hallmark of my Simple Heart Cure Diet, and it is no longer the linchpin of most diets, including Weight Watchers, which rebranded itself as WW in part to distance itself from the calorie-counting mentality. But, for many people, monitoring what they eat is a very important way to keep on track. Eating 1,200 calories per day would be a great weight-loss tactic.

DR. CRANDALL'S MOTIVATIONAL TIP
Focus on the Goal of Overall Health

Rather than looking at my plan as a restrictive diet only to lose weight (which never works long term!), focus on the long-term goal of improving your heart health and therefore your overall well-being. In the meantime, you'll probably lose weight. But it is better to focus on "winning," not just "losing."

PART TWO

The Simple Heart Cure Diet Lifestyle

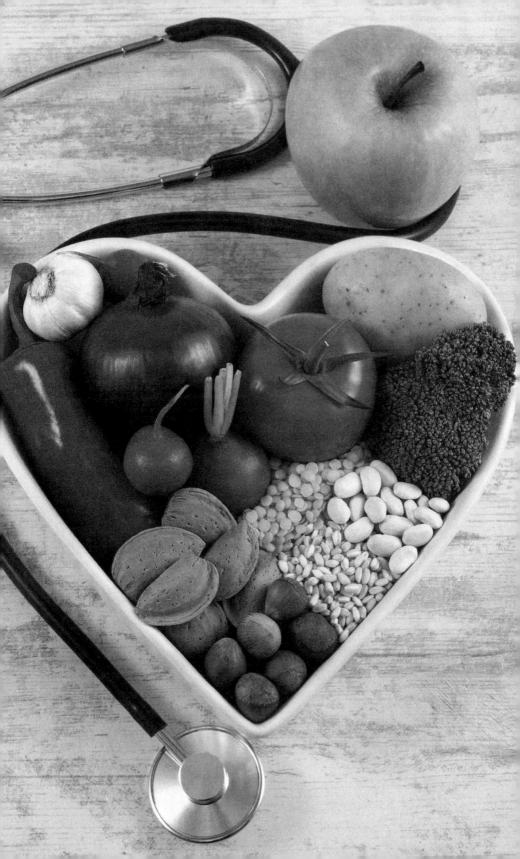

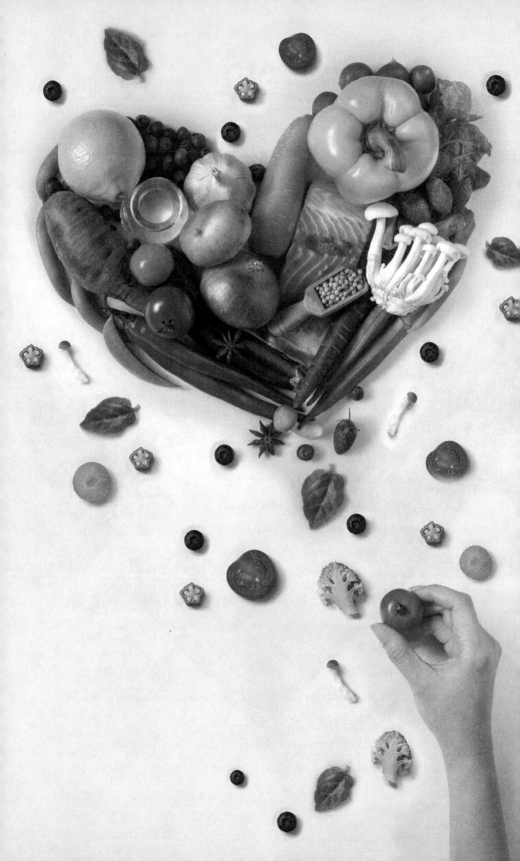

CHAPTER 5

The Simple Heart Cure Diet Food List

The foods in this chapter are the main items that comprise the Simple Heart Cure Diet. These foods are part of a plant-based diet that will make your cholesterol levels plummet, help you lose weight fast, and normalize your blood pressure and blood sugar levels. This list of food choices may be familiar from other popular vegetarian or plant-based eating plans because, basically, eating this way works! The "special recipes" in this book have their ingredients listed in each recipe individually.

Vegetables

This list includes all green leafy vegetables, string beans, asparagus, carrots, mushrooms, and tomatoes. Basically, if it's a vegetable, I encourage you to eat it. The only exceptions are avocados and olives, which are high in fat. Tomato sauce and tomato paste are also allowed but, again, when it comes to tomato sauce, check for added sodium or sugar; the fewer ingredients, the better.

Fruits

As with vegetables, the Simple Heart Cure Diet includes all fruits, including apples, banana, blueberries, cherries, cranberries, and so on, all the way to watermelons. For the sake of variety, I also include some unusual fruits, such as litchi nuts, although these must be fresh, not canned. In addition, I also allow some dried fruits, as long as they are not processed with added sugar. These include cherries, cranberries, dates, mango, papaya, and raisins. Of all of these fruits, the ones I recommend most are the berries because of their high antioxidant levels. Fruits such as apples and pears are very satisfying, and you can eat them with the skin for added fiber. Frozen fruits are fine as well; in fact, frozen blueberries or mango chunks, eaten almost straight from the freezer, make for a refreshing treat and dessert. Make sure to choose organic when you can!

Grains and Cereals

Bread, bagels, English muffins, crackers, etc., must be 100% whole wheat or whole grain, with no sugar added. Again, you have to carefully read the labels. Other grains allowed include barley, brown rice, wild rice, buckwheat, bulgur, corn, corn tortillas, hominy grits, kasha, millet, oatmeal, and oats. Whole grain couscous is also a good choice. Quinoa, a grain that soaks up flavor, has become increasingly popular, and you can also eat products made with rye or spelt, and wheat tortillas.

Another grain that you can use like quinoa is farro, which has been catching on in popularity. This ancient grain is high in protein, fiber, B complex vitamins, magnesium, and vitamin E. It's also relatively low in gluten. And farro is light in calories; at 100 calories per cup, it's about half the calories as pasta.

When cooked, farro resembles barley, but with a chewier texture, so it is great for soups and stews, and it doesn't get soggy. Farro can be used in salads, or as a substitute for pasta or rice.

When it comes to cereals, oatmeal, which is a combination of soluble and insoluble fiber, is an excellent cholesterol fighter. Other good cereal types that are low in calories and high in fiber include Grape-Nuts, multigrain flakes (without sugar), shredded wheat, Wheatena, and Uncle Sam cereal. Again, make sure to read labels and make sure that what you're buying is made from 100% whole grain, with no added sugar or malt (which converts to sugar).

Legumes

These vegetable seeds include beans, peas, and lentils and are among the most versatile and nutritious foods available. They are typically low in fat, high in nutrients, and contain no cholesterol. They are a good source of protein, and they are packed with soluble and insoluble fiber. In fact, they are one of the superfoods that helps to lower cholesterol. Legumes include all types of beans, including black-eyed peas, chickpeas, lima beans, navy beans, kidney beans, and more. Legumes can be your best friends when it comes to lowering your cholesterol levels, and I find many ways to include them frequently in my diet.

Protein

If you are accustomed to eating a conventional Western style diet (North Americans, I am talking to you), you are no doubt convinced that you must get your protein from red meat, poultry, or fish. This is a key reason the United States has such high rates of heart disease. People in many other countries get their protein from other sources, yet they are not protein deficient. While you are getting your numbers down to your target level, it is important that you get your protein from these other sources. Legumes, as I just mentioned, are an important source of protein. The main part of my Simple Heart Cure Diet gets its protein from high-omega-3 egg whites, soy, and soy alternatives such as edamame, soy fat-free sausages, soy hot dogs, and tempeh, tofu, and oil-free veggie meat substitutes. And, speaking of meat substitutes, the number of products in this category has simply exploded. Nowadays, there are many different brands of burgers, meat-free crumbles, chicken alternatives—you name it! This has been a tremendous boon for all of us who want to eat a plant-based diet, and so I urge you to experiment with these products, and use them in recipes as well. But check the label and make sure you're not picking items with long lists of chemicals or unrecognizable ingredients. Also, watch out for added sodium and sugar.

Dairy and Dairy Substitutes

Dairy products can be another hidden source of fat that keeps your cholesterol levels too high. I recommend nonfat Greek yogurt, and if you do use other dairy products, such as cottage cheese, sour cream, or cream cheese, make sure they are organic and nonfat. There are other types of "milk" made from other substances that are allowed, including oats, rice, and soy; just make sure they are unsweetened. Coconut water is becoming increasingly popular; just make sure it isn't flavored with sugar. If you are vegan or lactose intolerant, there is a growing number of dairy-free or lactose-free alternatives. Again, watch out for added sugar.

Fats and Oils

Although the whole idea of the Simple Heart Cure Diet is to reduce the fats in your blood, there are some fats you may find useful, including nondairy salad dressing, fish oil, flaxseed oil, and nonstick cooking spray.

In particular, I find olive oil cooking spray a valuable ally in the kitchen! When using any oil, only very small amounts are needed. Other heart-healthy oils are canola, flaxseed, avocado, walnut, grapeseed, and sesame oil. These oils are low in saturated fat and high in monounsaturated and polyunsaturated fat, which are healthier for your heart. Steer clear of other oils, including palm oil and coconut oil. These tropical oils are saturated fats, and should be avoided, even though they are often promoted as "heart healthy."

Herbs and Spices

Living the Simple Heart Cure Diet lifestyle requires you to give up your salt shaker, because salt can raise blood pressure. But if you get to know the wonderful array of herbs and spices you have available, you won't even miss it. This list includes flavor additives such as capers, chili flakes, fennel seeds, garlic, chili, green chilies, mace, mustard, natural vanilla, and pepper. Don't forget the vast array of fresh and dried herbs that are available to you. If you learn how to use herbs and spices well, your food will be bursting with both health and flavor.

Nuts

Add flavor to dishes with walnuts and almonds or snack on a small handful.

Sweeteners

Use small amounts of organic honey or pure maple syrup. These are better than refined "white sugar" because they contain some nutrients, such as magnesium, riboflavin, zinc, etc., and are not "empty calories." But keep the amounts small, like a dribble of honey on a bowl of oatmeal, for example.

DR. CRANDALL'S MOTIVATIONAL TIP

Slow and Steady

You'll have more success sticking to this way of eating if you gradually add in more plant-based proteins. The recipes in this book are a great start—and are so delicious that you won't feel deprived.

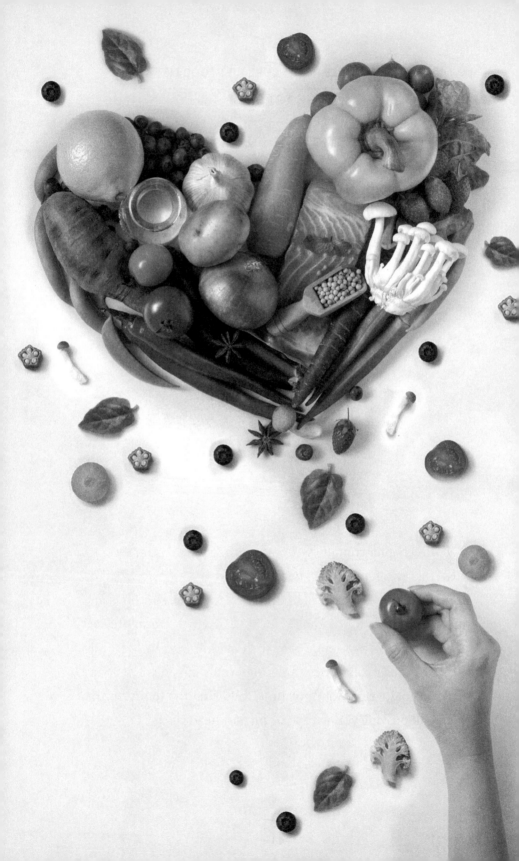

CHAPTER 6

The Simple Heart Cure Diet 28-Day Menu Plan

This chapter contains a month of Simple Heart Cure recipes that will jump-start your new heart-healthy lifestyle. You may also notice elsewhere in this book that some sections and recipes include foods that I do not list in the Simple Heart Cure Diet 28-Day Menu Plan, such as very lean turkey or an occasional egg yolk. These are foods you can add when you're at your goal weight, but, for now, following the foods on this plan will provide you with your biggest head start.

The Simple Heart Cure Diet Shopping List

In this shopping list, you'll find ingredients for the four-week Simple Heart Cure Menu Plan that follows. Many of the ingredients, such as the herbs and spices, you already have on hand. If you want to try all of the suggested recipes, these are the ingredients they contain. Remember, choose organic foods whenever possible, and always use real foods—nothing artificial or fake!

Week One

- Almond milk (unsweetened)
- Apples
- Baby carrots
- Balsamic vinegar
- Banana
- Basil leaves (fresh)
- Bell peppers
- Black pepper
- Blueberries (fresh or frozen is fine)
- Broccoli
- Brussels sprouts
- Cannellini beans
- Cantaloupe
- Carrots
- Celery
- Cherry tomatoes
- Cilantro
- Cinnamon
- Cucumber
- Cumin
- Dates
- Dill pickle
- Dried mint
- Eggplant

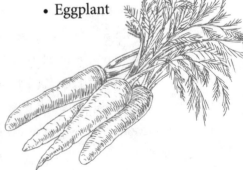

- Garbanzo beans
- Garlic
- Grape juice (organic)
- High-omega-3 eggs
- Honey
- Kidney beans
- Lemon (for juice)
- Lettuce
- Mango (fresh or frozen)
- Mint leaves (fresh)
- Mushrooms
- Nonfat Greek yogurt
- Nonfat herb and chive cream cheese
- Oatmeal (old-fashioned type, not instant)
- Olive oil cooking spray
- Onion

- Plum tomatoes
- Portabella mushrooms
- Potato
- Quinoa
- Raisins
- Red onion
- Red wine (low alcohol content)
- Red wine vinegar
- Scallions
- Shredded wheat (no added sugar)
- Spinach
- Strawberries
- String beans (whole)
- Sweet potato
- Tofu
- Tomatoes
- Veggie burger (oil-free)
- Walnuts
- WASA crackers
- Watermelon
- Whole wheat or whole grain sugar-free bread
- Wine vinegar
- Nonfat cream cheese

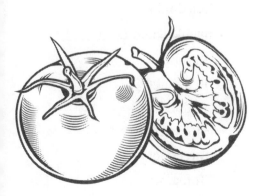

Week Two

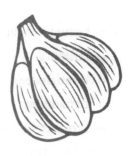

- Almond milk (unsweetened)
- Balsamic vinegar
- Banana
- Basil (fresh)
- Bell pepper
- Black beans
- Black pepper
- Blueberries
- Broccoli
- Brown rice
- Cayenne pepper
- Celery
- Cilantro
- Cinnamon
- Cucumber
- Cumin
- Dried cranberries
- Frozen vegetables (organic peas, corn, beans, or carrots)
- Garlic
- Green onions (also known as scallions)
- High-omega-3 eggs
- Honeydew melon
- Lemon (for juice)
- Lentils
- Mango
- Mesclun greens
- Navel orange
- Nonfat cottage cheese
- Nonfat Greek yogurt
- Oatmeal (old-fashioned type, not instant)
- Olive oil cooking spray
- Papaya
- Peaches
- Pear
- Plum tomatoes
- Raspberries
- Red onion
- Scallions
- Strawberries
- Sweet potatoes
- Tomatoes
- Vanilla extract

- Veggie burger (oil-free)
- Walnuts
- Whole wheat or whole grain pasta
- Whole grain penne pasta
- Whole wheat sugar-free bread
- Whole wheat sugar-free English muffin

Week Three

- Artichoke
- Bananas
- Basil
- Blueberries
- Brown rice
- Canned crabmeat
- Cantaloupe
- Carrot
- Cereal nuggets (i.e. Grape-Nuts)
- Chia seeds
- Chicken or vegetable broth
- Cilantro
- Cinnamon
- Cottage cheese (low-fat or fat-free)
- Crushed red pepper flakes
- Cucumber
- Dark chocolate (at least 70%)
- Eggplant
- Farro
- Feta cheese
- Flax seeds
- Fresh grapefruit
- Garlic (whole or grated)
- Garlic powder
- Greek yogurt
- Ground cumin
- Ground turkey
- High-omega-3 eggs
- Kalamata olives
- Lemon juice

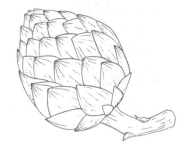

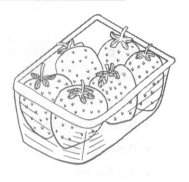

- Lime juice
- Low-sodium soy sauce
- Low-carb pita
- Low-carb tortillas
- Maple syrup
- Meat-free crumbles
- Mexican shredded cheese
- Navy beans
- Olive oil cooking spray
- Onion powder
- Orange
- Oregano
- Paprika
- Parmesan cheese (grated)
- Pizza sauce
- Portobello mushroom (large)
- Red or green bell peppers
- Rice vinegar
- Rolled oats
- Sage
- Salmon
- Scallions
- Sesame oil
- Sliced almonds
- Smoked salmon
- Spinach
- Strawberries
- Taco seasoning
- Thyme
- Tomato
- Tomato sauce (sugar-free)
- Tomatoes
- Turkey bacon
- Unsweetened almond milk
- Vanilla extract
- Whole wheat bread
- Whole wheat bread crumbs
- Whole wheat prebaked pizza crust
- Wild rice
- Zucchini

Week Four

- Asparagus spears
- Baby kale
- Balsamic vinegar
- Basil
- Blueberries
- Brown rice
- Chia seeds
- Chicken (shredded)
- Chives
- Cilantro
- Cinnamon
- Dark chocolate (at least 70% percent)
- Extra virgin olive oil
- Flax seeds
- Grape-Nuts (or similar nugget like cereal)
- High-omega-3 eggs
- Lime juice
- Low-carb tortillas
- Low-fat cheddar cheese
- Low-fat milk (or soy milk or almond milk)
- Low-fat shredded mozzarella cheese
- Maple syrup
- Meat-free "beef" crumbles
- Meat-free "chicken" patties
- Oranges
- Parsley
- Plain Greek yogurt
- Portobello mushroom (large)
- Quinoa
- Raspberries
- Rolled oats
- Skinless chicken wings
- Sliced almonds
- Spinach
- Spiral zucchini "noodles" (zoodles)
- Strawberries
- Peanut butter (Peanut butter usually has a very small amount of

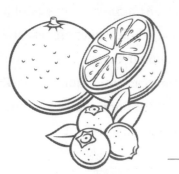

naturally occurring
sugar, but steer clear of
"low fat peanut butter,"
which sometimes has
added sugar.)
- Thyme
- Tomatoes

- Turkey bacon
- WASA crackers
- Whole garlic
- Whole grain hamburger
  bun
- Whole grain waffles

Your All-Important Breakfast

I always recommend that my patients start the day with what
I've come to call Dr. Crandall's Favorite Breakfast. Don't be
surprised, though, if you end up enjoying my favorite breakfast
two or three times a week, and eventually all of the time. Many
of my patients do, and I do too!

You can end your meals with coffee or tea. Coffee can be
lightened with a splash of almond milk, if you like.

The following pages will provide suggestions for designing
your Simple Heart Cure lifestyle for eating. Note that the rule
of thumb is to try to include protein at every meal to stave off
hunger. It doesn't matter which protein you eat, as long as you
avoid red meats, full-fat dairy, chemical additives, and added
salts and sugars. As you've read in previous pages, I've provided
suggestions for my favorite proteins. Aim for serving size of 3
ounces for fish, poultry, and plant-based meat alternatives, one
cup of your favorite beans (rinse canned beans in cold water
to reduce added salt), not more than one cup of nonfat Greek
yogurt or plant-based yogurt (no added sugar please!). If you
don't see a protein with a meal suggestion, feel free to add it.

♥ WEEK ONE ♥

Monday

BREAKFAST

- Scrambled eggs and whole wheat sugar-free toast
  Quick Recipe: Scramble three high-omega-3 egg whites in a nonstick pan that you've coated lightly with an olive oil cooking spray.
- ½ cup fresh blueberries

LUNCH

- Fresh spinach salad
  Quick Recipe: Toss spinach leaves with vegetables such as sliced mushrooms, chopped carrot, and chopped apple, and toss in a few raisins and walnuts as well.
- 2 WASA crackers topped with nonfat, organic cream cheese

DINNER

- Bountiful roasted vegetables
  Quick Recipe: Cut or chop an assortment of any type of vegetables you want (zucchini, onion, bell peppers, and sweet potatoes are good examples) and place on a baking sheet that you've sprayed with a small amount of olive oil cooking spray. Add sprinkle of dried or fresh cut herbs of your choice, if you like. Spray a little of the cooking spray on top and bake at 400°F until the vegetables are tender.

- Side salad of lettuce, cucumber, and cherry tomatoes, dressed with balsamic vinegar
- Tofu slices in a bowl topped with cinnamon and walnuts covered with a small amount of real maple syrup

Tuesday

BREAKFAST

- Whole grain French toast topped with strawberries
  Quick Recipe: Soak one slice of sugar-free, whole grain bread in a bowl with three beaten high-omega-3 egg whites. You can add cinnamon or vanilla to the eggs if desired. Cook bread on a nonstick pan or a pan lightly coated with olive oil cooking spray. While the bread is cooking, pour the remaining eggs over the bread. Flip the bread and cook on the other side. Top with fresh strawberries and a small amount of real maple syrup.

LUNCH

- Mixed three bean salad
  Quick Recipe: Drain and rinse canned cannellini beans, kidney beans, and garbanzo beans. Add some chopped celery, parsley, and red onion. Toss with apple cider vinegar and a small amount of honey.

- ½ cup fresh pineapple topped with nonfat yogurt (you can mix in some vanilla and just a tiny bit of pure maple syrup if you'd like).

DINNER

- Grilled oil-free veggie burger served on whole wheat sugar-free bun topped with lettuce, tomato, and onion slice
- Sliced dill pickle
- One cup steamed carrots, lightly dusted with cinnamon

Wednesday

BREAKFAST

- 1 cup old-fashioned cooked oatmeal (never instant!) topped with five or six chopped almonds and/or one tablespoon greek yogurt for added protein
- ½ sliced banana and a splash of sugar free almond milk if desired

LUNCH

- Strawberry spinach salad
  Quick Recipe: Combine the spinach with sliced strawberries, and drizzle with a bit of balsamic vinegar and honey to sweeten.
- ½ cup nonfat Greek yogurt, topped with chunks of fresh or frozen mango

DINNER

- Bruschetta-topped whole grain toast
  Quick Recipe: Stir together chopped ripe plum tomatoes, a few chopped fresh basil leaves, a chopped garlic clove, and some olive oil to moisten the mix (but as sparingly as possible). Spoon the mixture on to toasted whole wheat sugar-free bread and slice into squares. Place the mixture on top just before serving so the toast doesn't get soggy.
- ½ cup nonfat cottage cheese topped with fresh or frozen peaches

Thursday

BREAKFAST

- Mexican-style omelet
  Quick Recipe: Brown chopped onions and peppers in a pan lightly sprayed with olive oil cooking spray. Scramble three high-omega-3 egg whites and add a pinch of cumin, a pinch of garlic powder, and a pinch of chopped cilantro. Serve folded in an organic, sugar-free corn tortilla.
- ½ cup fresh blueberries

LUNCH

- Quinoa black bean salad

  Quick Recipe: Cook quinoa according to the packaged instructions. In a bowl, combine one teaspoon olive oil, a squeeze of fresh lime juice, pinch of cumin, ground coriander, fresh cilantro, minced scallions, diced tomatoes, and sliced bell pepper. Stir in drained, canned black beans. Mix with the cooled quinoa.

DINNER

- Greek tofu salad

  Quick Recipe: Cut firm tofu into chunks the size of dice and press them with paper towels to absorb any water. Steam the tofu for five 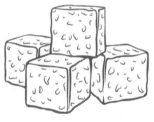 *minutes. Whisk together a small amount of olive oil, wine vinegar, basil, black pepper, oregano, and salt. Pour this mixture over the tofu and let it marinate. Meanwhile, chop up some fresh tomato, cucumber, and red onions and toss together with the chunks of tofu.*

- ½ cup low-fat yogurt topped with chopped dates and raisins and dusted with cinnamon

Friday

BREAKFAST

- 1 cup sugar-free shredded wheat with one sliced banana, 5 or 6 almonds, chopped, and unsweetened almond milk

LUNCH

- Cold asparagus salad with basil and tomatoes
  Quick Recipe: *Quickly cook whole string beans lightly so they are still crunchy, not limp. Drain and refrigerate until cold. Lightly sprinkle them with a bit of olive oil and red wine vinegar and serve the asparagus over large slices of ripe tomato. Top with fresh basil leaves.*
- ½ cup fresh cantaloupe

DINNER

- Baked potato topped with nonfat organic sour cream (or nonfat Greek yogurt) and chives
- 1 cup roasted brussels sprouts with balsamic vinegar
  Quick Recipe: *Slice fresh brussels sprouts in half, place them in a single layer on a baking pan sprayed with olive oil cooking spray, and drizzle the balsamic vinegar over them and make sure they are coated. Bake for 20 minutes at 375°F.*

Saturday

BREAKFAST

- Scrambled eggs with baked home fries
  Quick Recipe: Cut up small potatoes, spread them on a cooking sheet coated with a small amount of olive oil cooking spray, and lightly spray them again with cooking spray. Dust with pepper if you wish. Bake in a preheated oven at 475°F for 15–20 minutes or until tender but crispy.
- ½ cup fresh mango chunks
- 1 slice whole wheat sugar-free toast

LUNCH

- Nonfat cottage cheese with sliced cucumbers and tomatoes
- 1 slice sugar-free whole wheat bread spread with nonfat herb and garlic cream cheese
- 1 cup steamed broccoli tossed with minced garlic and a squeeze of lemon juice

DINNER

- Portobello basil sandwich

  Quick Recipe: *Stir lemon juice and nonfat Greek yogurt into a bowl, and brush over the sides of a large 4-ounce mushroom cap (stem removed, cap sliced). Grill or broil the mushroom until tender (2–3 minutes). Toast two slices of whole wheat sugar-free bread under the broiler. Spread half of the lemon juice/yogurt mixture on the toasted bread and arrange fresh basil leaves and sliced tomatoes on top of the grilled mushroom. Cut and serve.*

Sunday

BREAKFAST

- Banana omelet

  Quick Recipe: *Scramble three high-omega-3 egg whites and pour into a pan sprayed with olive oil. Cook as you would an omelet. Before you flip it, cover with banana slices. Top with cinnamon.*

- ½ cup fresh strawberries

LUNCH

- Watermelon salad

  Quick Recipe: *Arrange ½ cup watermelon, balled or cut into chunks, on a plate. Top with ½ cup fresh mint leaves and baby greens.*

- 2 WASA crackers topped with nonfat cream cheese and dusted with cinnamon

DINNER

- Grilled tofu salad with veggies
  Quick Recipe: *Grill the tofu and slice. Place 1 cup arugula, 1 tablespoon balsamic vinegar, ½ cup chopped onions, a quartered red tomato, ½ cup raw carrots, and a diced small cucumber in a bowl. Top with slices of grilled tofu and drizzle with balsamic vinegar.*

SNACKS

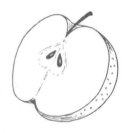

On my Simple Heart Cure Menu Plan, you can have snacks. Enjoy fruits and vegetables in their fresh, natural state or, if you prefer, jazz them up. Here are some ideas to get you started:

- Orange with mint. Peel and cut up an orange and combine with chopped mint
- Two dates with a cup of tea
- A small glass of low-alcohol red wine or organic grape juice, two WASA crackers and a handful of grapes
- Apple slices dusted with cinnamon
- ½ cup nonfat Greek yogurt with fresh raspberries stirred in
- Carrot sticks and 2 tablespoons hummus (watch the added salt if store-bought)
- Not more than 1/2 cup of chick peas, roasted with bit of olive oil spray

- Celery sticks or bell pepper wedges stuffed with organic nonfat organic cottage cheese and chopped chives
- Two WASA crackers topped with nonfat organic cream cheese
- Two dates stuffed with softened nonfat cream cheese
- Tofu slices in a bowl topped with cinnamon and walnuts covered with a small amount of real maple syrup. (This is my favorite dessert, and it also makes a great snack!)

♥ WEEK TWO ♥

Monday

BREAKFAST
- Scrambled eggs and cottage cheese omelet
  Quick Recipe: Pour three beaten high-omega-3 egg whites in a nonstick pan that you've coated lightly with olive oil cooking spray. When the eggs begin to thicken slightly, spoon in 1 or 2 tablespoons of nonfat organic cottage cheese. Flip over omelet style, dust with cinnamon, and serve.
- ½ cup fresh berries (any type)

LUNCH

- Sicilian salad
  Quick Recipe: *Peel and slice one large navel orange and arrange on plate, alternating with slices of red onion. Sprinkle with basil leaves and walnuts and drizzle with a tiny amount of balsamic vinegar. Sprinkle with pepper.*
- 1 slice sugar-free whole wheat toast
- ½ cup blueberries

DINNER

- Black beans and brown rice
  Quick Recipe: *Cook the brown rice and heat a can of drained black beans. Chop up some onion and carrots; red, yellow, or green peppers and some broccoli; chopped cilantro; a teaspoon of ground cumin; and a pinch of cayenne pepper. Cook the chopped vegetables, add the spices, and add the beans. Spoon it over the rice.*
- Chunks of melon with sliced strawberries

Tuesday

BREAKFAST

- 1 cup nonfat cottage cheese served with 1 cup fresh berries (any type or mix of berries, such as blueberries, raspberries, strawberries, and blackberries)
- 1 slice sugar-free whole wheat toast

LUNCH

- Rainbow fruit salad
  Quick Recipe: Blend 1 cup nonfat Greek yogurt with ½ ripe banana and a squeeze of lemon juice. Cut up a papaya, a mango, and a pear. Pour the yogurt dressing over the fruit.
- 2 WASA crackers

DINNER

- Roasted beets and sweet potatoes
  Quick Recipe: Cut beets and sweet potatoes into one-inch cubes. Arrange them on a baking pan lined with aluminum foil and coated with cooking spray, then spray them on top with cooking spray. Bake until tender (about 35 minutes).
- ½ cup nonfat Greek yogurt mixed with blueberries and strawberries

Wednesday

BREAKFAST

- Veggie scrambled eggs
  Quick Recipe: Beat three high-omega-3 egg whites. Add an assortment of chopped vegetables, such as spinach, green and red peppers, mushrooms, and onions—whatever veggies are on hand. Scramble and serve.
- 1 slice whole wheat sugar-free bread, toasted
- ½ cup fresh cherries

LUNCH

- Oil-free veggie burger topped with oven-roasted peppers
  Quick Recipe: *Place a whole red or green pepper on a baking sheet and broil until the skin has turned black and blistery. Remove from the oven and place the peppers into an airtight container, such as a paper or plastic bag or covered bowl. Wait 10–15 minutes, then remove and slide off the skin. Cut the pepper in half, remove the core and seeds, and slice into strips to top your burger.*
- Small green salad of spinach, lettuce, cucumber, and tomato dressed with red wine or balsamic vinegar

DINNER

- Veggie stuffed sweet potato
  Quick Recipe: *Bake one sweet potato, then cut off the top and scoop out the inside without breaking the skin. Mash the inside of the potato in a bowl. Stir in thawed frozen organic peas, corn, beans, and carrots—any small vegetable pieces you like. Re-stuff the potato skin and return to the oven for 15 minutes to brown.*
- ½ cup fat free Greek yogurt with raspberries and sliced banana

Thursday

BREAKFAST

- Whole grain French toast with blueberry compote
  Quick Recipe: Prepare the whole grain French toast according to the directions in Week One. To make the compote, place 1 cup fresh blueberries and 1 teaspoon vanilla extract in a pan and cook gently over low heat for 15 minutes.

LUNCH

- Lentil salad
  Quick Recipe: Take 1 cup chilled, steamed lentils and toss with chopped red peppers, cubed cucumber, and diced red onions. Toss with balsamic vinegar and dust with pepper if desired.
- 2 WASA Crackers

DINNER

- Whole wheat or whole grain pasta primavera
  Quick Recipe: Prepare pasta according to package instructions. Heat a nonstick skillet and add a little water to prevent sticking when you sauté. Sauté some diced bell pepper, onion, garlic cloves, tomatoes, and scallions. Add to the just-cooked pasta, stir, and serve.

Friday

BREAKFAST

- Scrambled eggs with browned onions and peppers
  Quick recipe: Beat three high-omega-3 egg whites in a bowl and set aside. Spray a nonstick skillet with a small amount of olive oil cooking spray and heat it until it's hot, then add chopped onions. Brown the onions, stirring constantly to prevent burning, until they are caramelized. Add some diced green peppers and cook until tender, then pour on the egg whites and scramble in the pan.
- Whole wheat English muffin (sugar-free)

LUNCH

- Indian cucumber and yogurt salad
  Quick Recipe: Peel and remove the seeds from one cucumber and thinly slice. Mix with one clove chopped garlic. Pour off any liquid that has formed and mix in 1 tablespoon dried mint. Beat nonfat plain yogurt until smooth, pour over cucumber mixture, and refrigerate. Serve over lettuce.
- Veggie burger with oven-baked "French fries"
  Quick Recipe: Slice one potato into strips. Arrange on baking sheet coated with a very small amount of olive oil cooking spray. Spray the potato strips with the cooking spray. Bake at 450°F for 30 minutes or until golden. Sprinkle with pepper if desired.

DINNER

- Roasted eggplant and chick peas with lemon
  Quick Recipe: Coat a baking pan with cooking spray. Slice and quarter an eggplant and place on the baking sheet, skin side down. Add ½ cup of drained canned chick peas. Spray with a small amount of cooking spray. Roast in the oven at 400°F until softened and brown. Remove from the oven and sprinkle with lemon juice.
- Steamed baby carrots dusted with cinnamon
- One 6-ounce glass of low-alcohol red wine or organic grape juice

Saturday

BREAKFAST

- Apple cinnamon oatmeal with almonds or walnuts
  Quick Recipe: In a small pot, add ¼ cup water, ½ chopped apple, a small handful of raisins, 1 teaspoon of vanilla, and cinnamon and simmer until the apple is soft. Cook your oatmeal as usual and combine with the fruit mixture. Top with 5-6 toasted almonds or walnuts, roughly chopped. Add a splash of almond milk if desired.

LUNCH

- Quinoa salad with dried fruits
  Quick Recipe: Cook quinoa until it is tender. Add some chopped celery, chopped green onions, raisins, dried cranberries, a splash of distilled white vinegar, a splash of lemon juice, and a pinch of cayenne pepper; mix together. Let it stand at room temperature before serving.

DINNER

- Whole wheat or whole grain penne with broccoli
  Quick Recipe: Prepare the penne according to the package directions. Cut 1 bunch of broccoli into florets, and, when 3 minutes of cooking time remain for the pasta, add the broccoli. Remove from the heat, drain pasta and broccoli, and return to pot, stir in some fresh halved cherry tomatoes and fresh basil leaves and serve.
- One 6-ounce glass low-alcohol red wine or a small glass of organic grape juice.

Sunday

BREAKFAST

- Breakfast burrito

  Quick Recipe: Coat a nonstick pan with olive oil cooking spray. Mix three high-omega-3 egg whites (or the equivalent) into a bowl, and add 1 tablespoon chopped raw scallions, 1 tablespoon raw cilantro, and ½ cup black beans. Scramble the egg mixture and then fold into a whole wheat or whole grain tortilla. Top with fresh chopped tomatoes and cilantro.

LUNCH

- Tomato salad with fresh greens

  Quick Recipe: Toss 1 cup fresh mesclun greens with two tablespoons red wine vinegar. Arrange the greens over sliced fresh tomatoes. Drizzle with a chive dressing made from fresh chopped chives mixed into nonfat yogurt.

- ½ cup nonfat cottage cheese with fresh peaches

DINNER

- Garden fresh cottage cheese salad with whole wheat or whole grain penne

  Quick Recipe: To nonfat cottage cheese, add chopped plum tomatoes, scallions, onions, and chopped peppers to taste, and sprinkle with pepper if desired. Serve with whole wheat or whole grain penne.

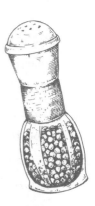

- Baked apple

  Quick Recipe: Hollow out one apple and squeeze a little lemon juice on the inside to prevent burning. Bake at 400°F for about 20 minutes. Sprinkle with cinnamon.

♥ WEEK THREE ♥

Monday

BREAKFAST

- Overnight oats

  Quick Recipe: Place ¼ cup uncooked rolled oats, ½ cup plain Greek yogurt, and 1 teaspoon chia or flax seeds into a bowl. Give them a good stir and refrigerate overnight (or at least 5 hours). In the morning, top with banana slices, any type of berries, or sliced almonds and dust with cinnamon.

- ½ whole grapefruit

LUNCH

- Farro Mediterranean salad

  Quick Recipe: Prepare farro according to package directions and put one portion aside to cool. In a bowl, mix together ½ cup diced cucumber, 1 cup diced tomato, minced Kalamata olives with pits removed, 2 ounces crumbled feta cheese, some minced scallions, and 2 teaspoons lemon juice (or to taste). Makes 2 servings.

- ½ cup strawberries topped with Greek yogurt and cinnamon

DINNER

- Roasted artichoke

  Quick Recipe: Preheat oven to 425°F. Trim a large artichoke by cutting off the stem and one inch off the top, and any pointy looking places on the leaves. Place artichoke stem-side down in a bowl and drizzle with lemon juice. Dust the artichoke with spices, such as thyme, oregano, or sage. Spray the artichoke with olive oil, wrap in aluminum foil, and bake until sizzling (1 hour, 20 minutes). Tip: Don't eat the leaves of the article, but nibble the soft base of each leaf, and eat the bottom with a knife and fork.

Tuesday

BREAKFAST

- Oatmeal pancake

  Quick Recipe: *Heat a spray-coated griddle or small pan over medium-high heat. Combine ½ cup rolled oats, ½ teaspoon vanilla, ½ teaspoon cinnamon, and an egg. Pour into the pan, shaping it as you would a pancake, cook for 2–3 minutes and flip. Top with 1 teaspoon of real maple syrup and half a banana, sliced.*

- ½ cup orange slices

LUNCH

- TLT (turkey, lettuce & tomato)

  Quick Recipe: *Spread two slices toasted whole wheat bread with mashed avocados. Then fill the sandwich with three slices of cooked turkey bacon, sliced tomatoes, and lettuce.*

- ½ cup diced cantaloupe and strawberries

DINNER

- Asian salmon

  Quick Recipe: Preheat oven to 350°F. Place one 6-ounce salmon filet, with skin on, in a small baking dish, which you've sprayed with cooking oil. Make an Asian marinade by combining ¼ cup low-sodium soy sauce with 1 teaspoon each of sesame oil, lemon juice, and rice vinegar. Cover the salmon with the marinade, adding more soy sauce if the fish isn't completely covered. Bake for 20 minutes, making sure the soy sauce mixture doesn't burn. Serve over brown or wild rice.

- ½ cup roasted or steamed brussels sprouts

Wednesday

BREAKFAST

- Blueberry smoothie bowl

  Quick Recipe: Peel ¼ banana, cut into chunks, and freeze. Place them in a blender, along with 1 teaspoon maple syrup, ¼ cup plain Greek yogurt, ½ cup unsweetened almond milk, ½ teaspoon vanilla extract, and two large ice cubes. Blend until smooth. Top with ¼ cup whole wheat flakes, ½ teaspoon sliced almonds, and ¼ cup fresh blueberries.

LUNCH

- Heart healthy taco salad

  Quick Recipe: *In a bowl, make a tossed salad, using any types of lettuces and greens you have on hand, or use a basic mix of romaine lettuce, diced plum or cherry tomatoes, and diced cucumber. Brown meatless crumbles, add about 1 teaspoon taco seasoning, and spoon atop the salad. Top with a small amount of Mexican shredded cheese. If you are watching your sodium, you can make taco seasoning without the salt that packaged mixes usually contain. In this case, make a seasoning by combining chili powder, ground cumin, paprika, crushed red pepper, garlic powder, onion powder, and dried oregano. You'll have plenty of flavor without adding salt.*

DINNER

- Spaghetti and meatballs

  Quick Recipe: *There are different ways to do healthy meatballs. My plan does allow for a limited amount of beef, so you can make them with chopped meat if you want. Ground turkey is another option, or you can now buy meat-free meatballs. If you're using lean ground beef or ground turkey, moisten with enough beaten egg to moisten, then add 1 teaspoon whole wheat bread crumbs,*

Parmesan cheese, parsley, and pepper. Brown the meatballs in a skillet and top with homemade or a healthy brand of jarred tomato sauce. Serve over whole wheat or whole grain spaghetti or farro.

- Tossed salad

Thursday

BREAKFAST

- Blueberry French toast

  Quick Recipe: *Whisk one or two eggs, then soak a slice of whole wheat bread or a low-carb tortilla or pita in the mixture. Sauté in a pan coated with olive oil cooking spray, and add ¼ cup low-fat or fat-free cottage cheese (whipped works particularly well) and about ⅓ cup fresh blueberries before flipping. Sprinkle on pumpkin or chia seeds. Dust with cinnamon.*

LUNCH

- Bruschetta

  Quick Recipe: *Dice one ripe tomato, and mix the pieces with a teaspoon of olive oil, a few leaves of chopped fresh basil, and some freshly grated garlic. Let sit for 10 minutes, and spoon onto slices of toasted or grilled whole wheat bread.*

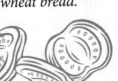

DINNER

- Citrus salmon

  Quick Recipe: Place ¼ cup orange juice, 1 chopped garlic clove, ¼ cup chicken or vegetable broth, and about 6 orange slices in a large sauté pan, cover and bring to a boil. Reduce heat to low and simmer, uncovered, for seven minutes. Add a salmon filet to this mixture and simmer 3–4 minutes until the salmon is opaque.

Friday

BREAKFAST

- Scrambled eggs and smoked salmon

  Quick Recipe: Pour a beaten whole egg or ½ cup egg whites into a nonstick pan that you've coated lightly with olive oil cooking spray. Add 2 ounces of smoked salmon pieces along with 2 teaspoons chopped scallops, and add it to the eggs.
- ½ cup fresh blueberries

LUNCH

- Crab-filled tomato

  Quick Recipe: First, make heart-healthy lump crab salad by combining canned crabmeat with lime juice, 2 tablespoons chopped onion, 1 tablespoon cilantro, and ¼ cup finely diced red or pepper. Use this crab salad to fill a hollowed out half tomato and serve.

DINNER

- Easy veggie pizza

  Quick Recipe: *Top a whole wheat, prebaked pizza crust with pizza sauce and top with shredded part-skim mozzarella cheese or other low- or no-fat cheeses. You can also top with any veggies you like—sliced bell peppers, mushrooms, zucchini slices, eggplant, etc. Place on a baking sheet. Brush the sides of the pizza lightly with olive oil. Bake at 450°F until the cheese melts.*

- 2 squares dark chocolate with tea

Saturday

BREAKFAST

- Blueberry pancake

  Quick Recipe: *Whisk one egg with 1½ tablespoons Greek yogurt (any flavor will also do, or you can use plain blended with 1 teaspoon maple syrup or honey). Mix well. Soak one low-carb tortilla or pita in the mixture, and add ⅓ cup blueberries. Cook in a skillet until the bottom is done, and then flip it over. Garnish with 1 tablespoon of yogurt in the center, ringed by a few fresh blueberries.*

LUNCH

- Turkey chopped salad

  Quick Recipe: *Chopped salads are very popular; they feature ingredients chopped into tiny pieces of uniform size. Almost any ingredients can be chopped; this one features sliced turkey (or meat-free luncheon meat), but you can use any lean meat as the main ingredient. Take any veggies you have on hand—lettuces, spinach, tomatoes, carrot strips. Chop them all together, along with 4 ounces cooked turkey. Then toss in other ingredients you may have as well, such as chickpeas, navy beans, crumbled feta, or hard cheese, and toss on top.*

DINNER

- Poached salmon

  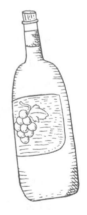

  Quick Recipe: *Heat ¼ cup lemon juice and ¼ cup water over medium heat in a large skillet for five minutes. Slice a 6-ounce piece of salmon into this poaching liquid and sprinkle with ½ teaspoon each dried parsley and chopped garlic, and add some black pepper. Bring to a slow boil and cook until salmon is firm (about 10–15 minutes).*

- Glass of low-alcohol red wine or organic grape juice

Sunday

BREAKFAST

- Quinoa fruit salad

  Quick Recipe: *Make an old-fashioned fruit salad, using fruits such as mango, pineapple, strawberries, and berries. Toss with ⅓ cup cooked quinoa in a bowl.*

- ½ cup plain Greek yogurt, sweetened with a bit of honey or maple syrup

LUNCH

- Avocado toast with turkey bacon

  Quick Recipe: *Prepare 4 slices of turkey or a veggie bacon substitute according to package directions. Mash ½ ripe avocado in a bowl and stir in 2 tablespoons lemon juice and a dash of cayenne pepper. Spread the avocado mixture on toasted whole wheat bread and top with the bacon and a ripe tomato slice.*

DINNER

- Stuffed mushroom caps

  Quick Recipe: *Rinse and drain four large mushrooms, taking off the stems and reserving the caps. Finely chop the stems. In a skillet, combine the stems, ⅓ cup meatless "sausage" crumbles, 1 tablespoon sliced green onions, 1 tablespoon water, and ¼ teaspoon minced garlic.*

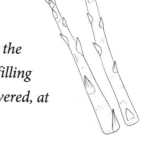

Cook covered, over medium-high heat for 4 minutes. Stir for about a minute more. Remove from heat, and arrange the mushrooms in a baking pan. Add the filling to the mushroom caps and bake, uncovered, at 425°F until heated. Serve warm.

- ½ cup asparagus spears

♥ WEEK FOUR ♥

Monday

BREAKFAST

- Muesli-topped Greek yogurt

  Quick Recipe: *Muesli can be eaten with milk or used as a topping for yogurt or fruit. To make it, preheat the oven to 400°F, and line a baking sheet with foil. Create a mixture of about ½ cup rolled oats, ½ cup nut-like cereal nuggets (Grape-Nuts or similar), ¼ cup sliced almonds, and 1 tablespoon flax seeds. Mix together ½ tablespoon olive oil and a teaspoon of honey. Pour over the oat mixture and toss to coat evenly. Bake 10–12 minutes, until toasted.*

LUNCH

- Baked portobello mushroom

  Quick Recipe: Brush off the dirt and cut off the stem of a large Portobello mushroom, then remove the "gills" and scrape the inside surface lightly so it is smooth. Brush both sides of the mushroom lightly with olive oil. Place on a baking dish with the cap side up and bake at 425°F for about 20 minutes or until soft and tender.

- Tossed salad

DINNER

- "Chicken" parmesan

  Quick Recipe: Sauté two meatless "chicken" patties in a pan. When the chicken patty is cooked, top with a simple healthy jarred or homemade tomato sauce and add some shredded low-fat mozzarella cheese. Cover briefly for a few moments so the sauce heats and the cheese melts, but be sure the patty doesn't burn. Serve with whole wheat or whole grain pasta.

Tuesday

BREAKFAST

- Breakfast tortilla

  Quick Recipe: Spray a pan with cooking spray. Add a low-carb tortilla and a layer of cooked spinach. Top with a scrambled egg.

LUNCH

- Sloppy Joe

  Quick Recipe: Make one serving of meatless crumbles in a skillet coated with cooking spray, add about 1 tablespoon of ketchup, some chopped onion and green pepper, and a dash of black pepper, and stir until cooked. Spoon over a whole wheat hamburger bun. This is also a tasty dish when the Sloppy Joe mixture is served over brown rice.

DINNER

- Roasted brussels sprouts with salmon

  Quick Recipe: Cut ½ pound of brussels sprouts in half and remove the stems. Cut up 3 oz salmon filet into chunks. Toss them with two tablespoons extra virgin olive oil. Sprinkle on ½ teaspoon of pepper. Place on a baking sheet and place in a preheated oven at 425°F for 20 minutes. Toss with 1 tablespoon Balsamic vinegar before eating.

Wednesday

BREAKFAST

- Quinoa porridge
  Quick Recipe: *Cook quinoa in milk (low-fat cow, soy, or almond) instead of water, and add cinnamon. Top with fresh fruit or a few squares of dark chocolate and some raspberries.*

LUNCH

- Muffin quiche
  Quick Recipe: *Preheat oven to 375°F. Coat a six-muffin tin with cooking spray or use paper liners. Crack six eggs into a bowl and whisk until smooth. Add ½ cup cooked spinach, ⅓ cup cooked turkey bacon and ⅓ cup low-fat shredded cheddar cheese. Bake until the eggs set (about 15–20 minutes). Refrigerate extra "quiches" for meals later in the week.*
- Baked apple

DINNER

- Baked chicken wings and sweet potato "fries"
  Quick Recipe: *Combine 1–2 tablespoons olive oil, 1 teaspoon garlic powder, 1 teaspoon chili powder, and a pinch of black pepper in a plastic bag; seal and shake. Add*

five skinless chicken wings, reseal, and shake some more. Cut up 4 ounces peeled sweet potato into "fries" and place wings on one side of sheet pan, with sweet potato on other side. Spray sweet potato lightly with olive oil. Bake the wings and sweet potato in a preheated oven at 375°F for an hour, or until cooked through.

Thursday

BREAKFAST

- Red-white-and-blue parfait
  Quick Recipe: Alternate layers of fresh blueberries and sliced strawberries, separating them with a layer of plain Greek yogurt. You can drizzle the layers with a bit of honey or maple syrup for sweetness. Sprinkle the top with cinnamon and chia seeds.

LUNCH

- Spiral zucchini parmesan
  Quick Recipe: Buy frozen spiral zucchini noodles and make according to the package directions. Drizzle on 1 teaspoon of olive oil and sprinkle with Parmesan cheese.
- Greek salad

DINNER

- Roasted asparagus with almonds
  Quick Recipe: Cut the ends off of ½ pound fresh asparagus spears. Place on a baking sheet, then toss with 1 tablespoon olive oil, and season with pepper and garlic powder. Roast until the asparagus is tender, place on plate, and top with toasted almonds.
- Baked salmon

Friday

BREAKFAST

- Savory oatmeal
  Quick Recipe: Prepare oatmeal as usual, but add a pinch of sea salt and pepper.

LUNCH

- Cottage cheese with diced cucumber and scallions
- Dark chocolate-dipped fruit
  Quick Recipe: Dip a variety of fruits (banana slices, strawberries, pineapple) into melted dark chocolate. Also makes a great party recipe.

DINNER

- Tofu vegetable stir-fry

  Quick Recipe: *Peel and slice a small onion. Chop 2 garlic cloves, ¼ cup carrots, ¼ cup bell peppers, and ½ cup broccoli florets. Cut ¼ pound firm tofu into squares, and set aside. Mix together 1 tablespoon low sodium soy sauce, 1 tablespoon olive oil, and 1 teaspoon sesame oil. Preheat a large sauté pan on high for 2–3 minutes. Add all ingredients and cook, stirring constantly, for about 10 minutes or until vegetables are tender.*

Saturday

BREAKFAST

- Peanut butter waffle

  Quick Recipe: *Take a cooked whole grain frozen waffle, and spread with two tablespoons of natural, sugar-free peanut butter. Top with sliced bananas and raisins.*

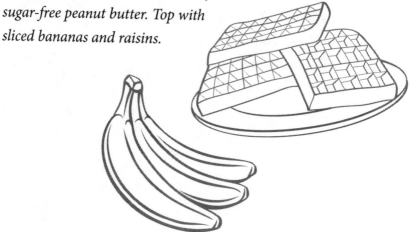

LUNCH

- Healthy Caesar salad

  Quick Recipe: *Make a healthy Caesar salad by blending until smooth ½ cup Greek yogurt, ¼ cup grated Parmesan cheese, 1 tablespoon extra virgin olive oil, 1 tablespoon lemon juice, 1 teaspoon Dijon mustard, ½ chopped garlic clove, and ½ teaspoon anchovy paste. Drizzle on a tossed salad and refrigerate the remainder.*
  Shred pieces of romaine lettuce, add grilled chicken or shrimp, and top with healthy Caesar dressing.

DINNER

- Garlic basil herb tomatoes

  Quick Recipe: *Cut a medium tomato into quarters and place on a baking sheet. Top with 1 chopped garlic clove, and bake at 400 F until softened. Place the tomato pieces in a serving bowl and top with 1 teaspoon each of fresh basil, parsley, and thyme and add a dash of pepper. Top with crumbled feta cheese.*

Sunday

BREAKFAST

- Pumpkin oatmeal

  Quick Recipe: Combine 1 cup rolled oats and 1 cup unsweetened almond milk and stir over medium heat. Bring to a boil, until desired consistency is reached, and then stir in ⅛ cup canned pumpkin. Add a little maple syrup for sweetness if desired.

LUNCH

- Orange beet salad

  Quick Recipe: Whisk ⅛ cup lemon juice, 2 ounces baby kale, and 2 ounces precooked beets. Put this mixture on a plate, then top with ½ sliced avocado and ½ cup orange segments.
- 2 WASA crackers

DINNER

- Mexican chicken rollups

  Quick Recipe: Mash up an avocado along with 4 ounces shredded chicken, chopped bell pepper, 1 teaspoon chives, ½ teaspoon chopped cilantro, and ¼ cup low-fat cheddar cheese, and stir until combined. Spread the mixture on a low-carb tortilla. Add a squeeze of lime juice. Roll the tortilla up tightly, then cut off the end and slice into 1-inch rolls. Also makes a great party snack.

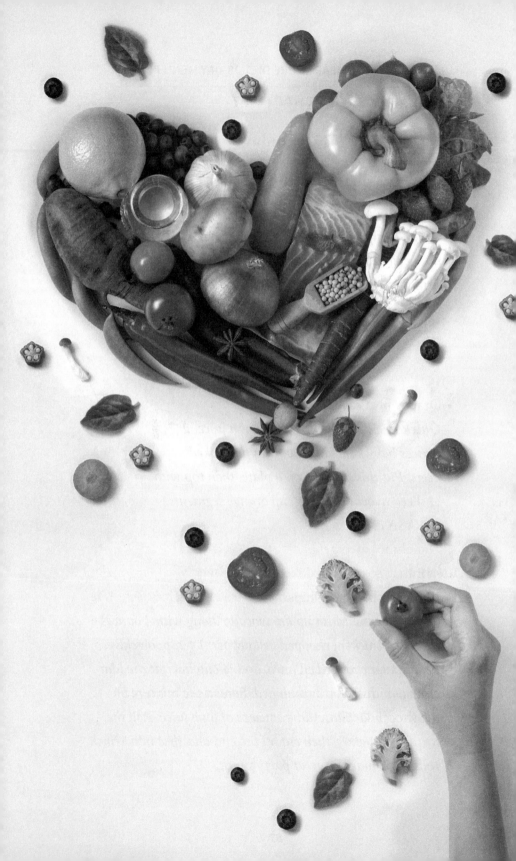

CHAPTER 7

The Simple Heart Cure Diet Special Recipes

Sometimes diets get boring, and variety is a great antidote for that, so registered dietitian Sue Gebo created a special set of recipes for this program that are a little more elaborate to make but are also low in fat, calories, and sugar. For those who want to try them, here are additional ingredients you may want to keep on hand—followed by the recipes. To avoid redundancy, this list includes ingredients not already included in the shopping list in Chapter 6.

Special Recipe Ingredients

Barley Risotto with Shiitake Mushrooms
- White wine, such as dry sherry (Don't buy "cooking wine," as it tends to be low quality.)
- Fresh or dried shiitake mushrooms
- Pearl barley
- Romano cheese

Spicy Cauliflower-Stuffed Peppers
- Long or small red bell peppers
- Frozen riced cauliflower
- Chili powder
- Cayenne pepper
- NoSalt (or other potassium-based salt substitute)

Rich Aquafaba Chocolate Mousse
- Canned low-sodium chickpeas
- Cream of tartar

Easy Barley Casserole
- Sliced fresh mushrooms or unsalted canned slices, stems, or pieces

Asian-Style Grilled Tofu
- Scallions

Chicken with Tomatoes and Fresh Herbs over Pasta
- Boneless chicken breast
- Fresh sage leaves
- Whole wheat pasta

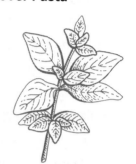

Asian Soup with Lean Pork Meatballs
- Boneless pork loin chops
- Green cabbage
- Dry sherry

Easy Microwave Polenta
- Stone ground, whole grain, yellow cornmeal

Italian-Style Spaghetti Squash Bake
- Spaghetti squash
- Part-skim or fat-free ricotta cheese

Taco Lasagna
- No-salt taco seasoning mix
- Salsa (see recipe if you wish to make your own)

Stroganoff Casserole
- Brown mushrooms, such as baby bella (crimini)
- Ground bison (if you wish an alternative to ground turkey)
- Dry red wine
- Light sour cream

Smoky Fish and Veggie Bowl

- Tinned fish, such as sardines or herring steaks or salmon
- Tomato paste in a tube
- Smoked paprika or liquid smoke

Indian-Style Egg Roll-Ups

- Low-sugar ketchup
- Apple cider vinegar, if preferred to rice vinegar
- Sriracha sauce
- Soft whole wheat tortilla, taco-size

Slow Cooker "Roast" Chicken

- 3–4-pound chicken
- Cornstarch

Quick Chicken Curry

- Nonfat evaporated milk or ½ cup light coconut milk
- Curry powder
- Unsalted roasted peanuts

Crustless Spinach Quiche

- Frozen spinach
- Skim milk
- Low-fat sharp cheddar cheese

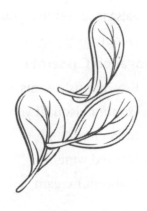

Microwave Eggplant Parmigiana

- Low-sodium marinara sauce

Asian Pork Tenderloin
- Pork tenderloin

Slow Cooker Spanish Rice
- Sodium-free beef flavor granulated bullion

Vegetarian West African Stew
- Canned small red beans
- Ground coriander
- Canned diced tomatoes with green chilies

Black Bean Quinoa Salad
- Sherry vinegar
- Chipotle pepper in adobo (smoked paprika may be substituted)
- Canned low-sodium black beans

Beet Brownies
- Unsweetened dark cocoa powder (Dutch processed)
- No-salt sliced beets, canned or jarred
- Dark brown sugar

THE RECIPES

BARLEY RISOTTO WITH SHIITAKE MUSHROOMS

Makes 7 servings

Per serving (1 cup)—269 calories

This delicious take on risotto incorporates barley, a great source of soluble fiber and a whole grain that is underutilized in North America. This dish also incorporates shiitake mushrooms, which contribute additional soluble fiber, as well as garlic and onions. It is quite filling, so it can be a satisfying main dish along with a salad.

- 5 cups low-sodium vegetable or chicken stock
- 1 cup white wine, such as dry sherry
- 1 tablespoon olive oil
- 1 cup thinly sliced shiitake mushrooms or 5 large dried shiitake mushrooms
- 1 medium onion, finely chopped
- 4 garlic cloves, pressed through garlic press
- 1½ cups pearl barley, rinsed
- ½ teaspoon black pepper
- ½ cup grated Romano cheese

1. Bring vegetable stock and wine to a boil. Turn off heat and keep covered.
2. If using dried shiitake mushrooms, place whole mushrooms in measuring cup with ½ cup water. Microwave on high for 1–2 minutes. Let cool. Drain, reserving mushroom broth and adding broth to warm stock. When the shiitake mushrooms are cool enough to handle, thinly slice them, discarding woody parts of stems.
3. Heat olive oil in a 3-quart Dutch oven or heavy pot. Sauté onion and garlic until soft. Add sliced shiitakes (if using fresh mushrooms, cook until most of the moisture has cooked off). Add barley and stir.
4. Add broth in 1-cup additions and cook over medium-high heat, stirring well after each addition until broth is mostly absorbed. Continuing adding stock in 1-cup increments, stirring after each addition until broth is mostly absorbed. After all broth has been added, cover and continue cooking over low heat until barley is tender, about 20 minutes, stirring often to prevent sticking.
5. Add Romano cheese and black pepper, stirring well.
6. Serve with additional black pepper and Romano, if desired.

SPICY CAULIFLOWER-STUFFED PEPPERS

Makes 8 servings

Per serving (1 stuffed pepper)—179 calories

- 4 long or 8 small red bell peppers
- 12 ounces frozen riced cauliflower, thawed
- 1 tablespoon olive oil
- 1 medium onion, chopped
- 2 garlic cloves, minced
- 1 pound 93% lean ground turkey
- 1 tablespoon chili powder
- 2 teaspoons smoked paprika
- 1 teaspoon ground cumin
- ½ teaspoon black pepper
- ½ teaspoon cayenne pepper (or more to taste)
- 1 teaspoon potassium-chloride-based salt substitute, such as NoSalt
- 8-ounce can no-salt tomato sauce
- ½ cup shredded part-skim mozzarella

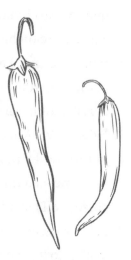

1. Prepare the peppers.
   a. If using long red peppers, slice in half crosswise to yield two pepper cups. Scoop out seeds and white parts of stem end.
   b. If using smaller, rounder peppers, slice off stem end and scoop out seeds. Cut flesh from the stems, chop, and add to chopped onion.

2. Stand pepper cups, cut side up, in a large microwaveable casserole or two 8 x 8-inch baking dishes. Microwave on high for 90 seconds to soften (If using two dishes, microwave each dish separately.) Remove from microwave and set aside.

3. In large skillet, heat ½ tablespoon olive oil over medium-high heat. Add thawed riced cauliflower and sauté until slightly softened. Remove from heat and place cauliflower in bowl. Wipe out skillet.

4. Return skillet to heat and add remaining ½ tablespoon oil. Add chopped onion (and chopped bell pepper, if using smaller peppers) and sauté until softened. Add garlic, ground turkey, salt substitute, and spices. Cook, stirring and chopping turkey into small pieces, until turkey is no longer pink.

5. Add tomato sauce and riced cauliflower. Stir to blend. Cook for 2–3 minutes.

6. Turn off heat. Divide filling among pepper cups, pressing to fill lobes in bottoms of peppers.

7. Sprinkle a little shredded mozzarella on top of each pepper.

8. Bake at 350°F oven for 20 minutes.*

   To cook in microwave, cook each dish at 100% power (high) for 2½ minutes and at 60% power (medium) for 5 minutes.

EGGPLANT STUFATO

Makes 4 servings

Per serving without cheese—104 calories

Per serving with 2 tablespoons shredded mozzarella—140 calories

This is an easy, tasty way to prepare eggplant without all the oil and breading. This "stew" makes a great side dish with grilled chicken or a filling main dish when served with a sprinkling of Parmesan and/or shredded part-skim mozzarella. Rich in anthocyanins and soluble fiber, eggplants are a worthy addition to a heart-healthy meal plan.

- 1 tablespoon olive oil
- 1 medium onion, coarsely chopped
- 1 garlic clove, sliced or minced
- 1 medium to large eggplant (Italian or globe), cut into ¾-inch cubes
- 2 medium fresh tomatoes, diced; or one 14.5-ounce can no-salt diced tomatoes
- ½ teaspoon crushed red pepper (optional)
- Potassium-chloride based salt substitute, such as NoSalt
- Freshly ground black pepper
- ½ cup Parmesan and/or shredded mozzarella (optional)

1. Heat olive oil in heavy pan (2–3 quarts) that is large enough to accommodate the cubed eggplant. The eggplant will shrink while cooking.

2. Add onion to the oil and sauté until softened.

3. Add garlic and cook briefly, stirring to prevent burning.

4. Add eggplant; sauté until cubes are covered with oil and slightly softened.

5. Add tomatoes, a sprinkle of salt substitute, and crushed red pepper, if using, and bring to a simmer. Cover and simmer over low heat until the eggplant is very soft, about 10 minutes.

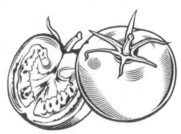

6. Season with salt substitute and black pepper to taste.

7. If using as a main dish, ladle into bowls and top with Parmesan and/or shredded part-skim mozzarella.

TOMATO AND PARMESAN BROWN RICE RISOTTO

Makes 4 servings

Per serving (1½ cups)—378 calories

This dish is delicious whether you use fresh cherry tomatoes in season or canned, no-salt diced tomatoes. The key to risotto is stirring while it cooks, which achieves a creamy texture. This risotto can be served as a main dish or as a side dish with grilled chicken.

- 5 cups low-sodium or no-salt chicken broth
- 2 tablespoons extra virgin olive oil
- 1 medium onion, finely chopped
- 3 garlic cloves, thinly sliced
- 1 tablespoon tomato paste
- 2 cups cherry tomatoes (cut them in half to avoid scalding your tongue when eating the risotto), or one 14.5-ounce can no-salt diced tomatoes (drain, saving juice—add the tomato juice to the chicken broth)
- 1 cup short grain brown rice (if not available, use long grain brown rice and extend the cooking time)
- Salt substitute, such as NoSalt
- ¾ cup finely grated Parmesan
- Freshly ground black pepper
- Fresh basil leaves, thinly sliced (optional)

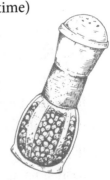

1. Bring broth to a simmer in a medium saucepan; keep warm over medium-low heat until ready to use.

2. Meanwhile, heat the olive oil in a large saucepan over medium heat. Add the onion and cook, stirring often, until golden and very soft, 8–10 minutes. Add garlic and cook, stirring, until softened, about 1 minute, taking care not to burn it. Add tomato paste and cook, stirring often, until it darkens and begins to stick to pan, about 2 minutes. Add tomatoes and cook, stirring occasionally, until steaming, about 2 minutes. (If using canned tomatoes, cook until heated through.)

3. Stir in rice; season with NoSalt, and reduce heat to medium-low. Cook, stirring, until some grains are translucent, about 5 minutes. Add 2 cups broth and simmer, stirring frequently, until completely absorbed, about 10 minutes. Add another 2 cups broth and continue to cook, stirring frequently, until rice is cooked through and most of the broth is absorbed, 15–20 minutes. Taste to see if texture of rice is soft enough to your liking. If not, turn off heat, cover tightly, and let sit for 10 minutes to complete cooking.

4. Add Parmesan and remaining 1 cup broth and cook, stirring, over medium-low heat until risotto is creamy looking, about 5 minutes. Season with more salt substitute if needed. Divide risotto among bowls. Top with black pepper and a dusting of Parmesan. Sprinkle with fresh basil, if using.

RICH AQUAFABA CHOCOLATE MOUSSE

Makes about 6 servings

Per serving (½ cup)—127 calories

This mousse is the most decadent, rich-tasting dessert! The texture is reminiscent of fluffy frosting. Instead of cream or eggs, it uses the liquid from a can of chickpeas, called aquafaba ("bean water"), which whips up like cream! Aquafaba is an almost flavorless liquid, so the chocolate in this recipe completely disguises this secret ingredient.

- 15.5-ounce can low-sodium chickpeas
- 5 ounces dark chocolate chips (about ⅔ cup) or 5-ounce dark bar chocolate
- ¼ teaspoon cream of tartar (to stabilize foam)

1. Place a small sieve over a 2½–3-quart bowl or the bowl of a stand mixer. Shake can of chickpeas before opening, then open the can. Pour chickpeas and all liquid from the can into the sieve and allow to drain for a few minutes. Shake strainer to drain out as much liquid as possible. Reserve chickpeas for another use. The liquid, called aquafaba, is what will make the mousse.

2. Cover bowl of aquafaba with a plate or plastic wrap. Place in the refrigerator for 20–30 minutes. Chilling the liquid will help it whip up faster.

3. Meanwhile, measure out the chocolate and place in a 1-cup microwave-safe measuring cup. If using bar chocolate, break up into small pieces.

4. Microwave on high for 20 to 30 seconds at a time, stirring after each interval, until most of the chocolate is melted, being careful not to burn. Stir with a fork or small whisk until all chocolate is melted and very smooth. Set aside to cool briefly.

5. Remove the bowl of aquafaba from the refrigerator. Add cream of tartar to the liquid. Using a handheld electric beater or a stand mixer, start at low speed to blend in the cream of tartar. After the cream of tartar is blended into the liquid, increase the speed little by little until you reach high speed. The mixture will become foamy, then thicker, and, finally, reach the consistency of whipped cream with stiff peaks. This may take as little as 3 minutes or as long as 5–7 minutes.

6. If using a hand mixer, turn off the mixer and add melted chocolate, all at once. Immediately resume beating at medium to medium-low speed until well blended and fluffy. If using a hand mixer, leave the mixer on at medium-low speed and pour in the melted chocolate and continue to beat until well blended.

7. Taste the mousse and decide if you want to add any flavoring, such as raspberry extract or other natural flavoring, or a little more sweetener, such as maple syrup or monk fruit extract. If you add ingredients, whip again until well blended.

8. Spoon mouse into ½-cup dessert dishes, such as 4-ounce ramekins. Cover dishes and chill for at least one hour.

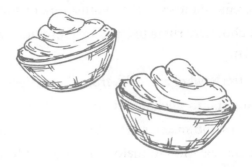

EASY BARLEY CASSEROLE

Makes 6 servings

Per serving—174 calories

Here's a tasty way to serve soluble-fiber-rich barley. Serve alongside grilled fish or chicken or grilled tofu slices with a salad or steamed veggies.

- 2 teaspoons olive oil
- 4 ounces sliced mushrooms or 8-ounce can no-salt-added mushrooms (sliced OR stems and pieces)
- ½ cup diced celery
- 1 medium onion, chopped
- 1 garlic clove, minced
- 14.5-ounce can diced tomatoes in juice or 1¾ cups chopped fresh tomatoes with their juice
- 1½ cups low-sodium chicken broth
- 1 cup barley
- ½ teaspoon black pepper
- 2 tablespoons Parmesan cheese
- 1 teaspoon fresh parsley, chopped

1. In 3-quart, microwave-safe covered casserole or a 3-quart microwave-safe bowl with microwave-safe plate to cover, combine olive oil, mushrooms, celery, onion, and garlic. Cover and cook in the microwave on high for 2–3 minutes.

2. Stir in tomatoes with juice, chicken broth, barley, and black pepper. Cover and cook on high for 5 minutes, stir, then cook another 5 minutes on high. Stir again and cook 10 minutes at 60% power (medium).

3. Sprinkle with Parmesan cheese and parsley, cover, and let stand 10 minutes before serving. Taste and adjust seasoning with salt substitute, lemon juice, or additional Parmesan cheese.

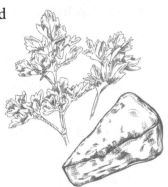

ASIAN-STYLE GRILLED TOFU

Makes 6 slices

Per slice—110 calories

This grilled tofu is great with stir-fried Asian-style veggies and steamed brown rice, but use your imagination! Pressing the tofu (step 2) increases uptake of the marinade for more flavor, and it encourages slices to crisp up when grilled. If using pre-pressed tofu, omit steps 2 and 3.

- 14-ounce to 16-ounce block firm or extra-firm tofu (or pre-pressed tofu)
- 1 tablespoon olive oil (not extra virgin)
- 1 thick slice fresh ginger, grated (2–3 tablespoons)
- 6–7 garlic cloves, pressed through garlic press
- 3 tablespoons reduced-sodium soy sauce
- 1 tablespoon pure maple syrup
- ¼–½ teaspoon black pepper
- ¼ teaspoon crushed red pepper flakes (optional)
- 1 scallion, thinly sliced (to garnish)

1. Open the package of tofu and drain. Slice tofu in half, then slice each half into 3 equal slices (about ¾ inch thick). If using pre-pressed tofu, jump to step 4.
2. Line a 9 x 13-inch baking dish with a clean kitchen towel or a double layer of paper towels. Lay tofu slices on their

wider sides in a single layer in an 8-inch square on top of towels in the center of the baking dish. Cover with another clean kitchen towel (or fold over the first towel to cover) or another double layer of paper towels. Top with an 8 x 8-inch inch baking dish so that bottom of the dish presses on all six tofu slices. Place a heavy pan, water-filled teakettle, or 2–3 heavy cans of food in the 8 x 8-inch dish to press tofu slices. Let sit for at least 30 minutes.

3. Remove the 8 x 8-inch dish from the top of the tofu and remove weights from the dish. Remove towel or paper towels from tofu.

4. Arrange the tofu in a single layer in the 8 x 8-inch baking dish. Using a fork, pierce each tofu slice deeply several times, stabilizing each slice with your free hand to avoid tearing. This step will enhance uptake of marinade.

5. In a 2-cup, microwave-safe measuring cup, place olive oil, ginger, and garlic. Microwave, uncovered, at 60% power (medium) for 2 minutes, stirring after 1 minute. Add reduced-sodium soy sauce, maple syrup, 5 tablespoons water, black pepper, and crushed red pepper, if using. Return to microwave and cook at 60% power (medium) for 2 more minutes.

6. Pour the hot marinade evenly over the tofu slices, then flip the slices over to cover both sides with marinade. Seal the dish with plastic wrap or cover with a well-fitting plate. Refrigerate for at least 6 hours, turning over the tofu slices occasionally to help absorb more of the marinade.

7. When ready to grill, preheat a nonstick grill pan or any nonstick pan over medium heat. Spray the pan with nonstick olive oil cooking spray, or brush the pan with olive oil. Remove the tofu slices from the dish and shake off excess marinade, but reserve the marinade. Grill slices until golden and crisp on one side (3–4 minutes), then flip and cook on the other side until golden.

8. Pour reserved marinade into a 2-cup, microwave-safe measuring cup. Heat in microwave at 60% power for 1–2 minutes, until bubbling. Stir in scallions. Use this sauce to top the tofu slices.

CHICKEN WITH TOMATOES AND FRESH HERBS OVER PASTA

Makes 4 servings

Per serving without cheese—376 calories

Add a tossed green salad and a glass of dry red wine for a Mediterranean treat!

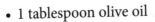

- 1 tablespoon olive oil
- 1 medium onion, chopped
- 1 small red pepper, finely chopped
- 1 can no-salt-added mushrooms, drained; or 1 cup fresh mushrooms, sliced
- 3 tablespoons dry red wine
- 14.5-ounce can no-salt diced tomatoes or 1¾ cups chopped fresh tomatoes
- 1 garlic clove, minced
- ½ teaspoon honey
- Potassium-chloride-based salt substitute, such as NoSalt
- Freshly ground black pepper
- 12 ounces boneless skinless chicken breast, cut into 1½-inch chunks; or 12 ounces (2–3) boneless skinless chicken thighs, cut into 1-inch chunks
- 1 tablespoon chopped fresh basil or 1 teaspoon dried basil
- ½ tablespoon chopped fresh parsley
- 1 tablespoon chopped fresh sage leaves (or ½ teaspoon dried—but fresh sage offers much more flavor to this dish)

- ½ pound whole wheat pasta

1. Heat the oil in a nonstick skillet. Sauté onion, pepper, and mushrooms until softened.
2. Add the wine; simmer for 2–3 minutes to allow alcohol to cook off.
3. Add the tomatoes with juice, garlic, honey, salt substitute, and pepper. Bring to a boil, reduce heat, and simmer, covered, for 15–20 minutes.
4. Add the chicken, stir well, cover, and simmer over low heat for another 10 minutes, checking chicken for doneness (no longer pink inside) after 10 minutes. If using chicken breast, take care not to overcook it or else it will become dry. If chicken is still pink inside, cook for a few more minutes.
5. Cook pasta to desired doneness while the sauce is cooking. Cooking pasta longer than the label suggests will render the pasta softer and silkier and will increase volume, but if you like it firm, follow label directions for *al dente*. Drain and rinse.
6. While pasta cooks, add herbs to the sauce, cover, and simmer for a few minutes to blend the flavors. Adjust seasoning with more black pepper and salt substitute.
7. Divide pasta and sauce among four bowls. Top with a sprinkling of Parmesan or Romano cheese and more freshly ground black pepper. Drizzle a little extra virgin olive oil over each serving, if desired.

ASIAN SOUP WITH LEAN PORK MEATBALLS

Makes 3 servings

Per serving without optional toppings—318 calories

This cozy soup makes a great light dinner for two. Boneless, trimmed pork loin chops are extremely lean. If you don't eat pork, substitute ground turkey. Using coleslaw mix in step 5 saves a few prep steps, but experiment, if you wish, with adding other chopped leafy greens or fresh baby spinach to the broth.

MEATBALLS:

- ½ pound boneless pork loin chops (2 small chops), trimmed of all fat and cut into half-inch cubes
- 3 garlic cloves, peeled
- 1 cup green cabbage, chopped
- 1 scallion, chopped
- 1 tablespoon grated ginger
- 1 tablespoon reduced-sodium soy sauce
- 1 tablespoon dry sherry
- ½ teaspoon toasted sesame oil
- ¼ teaspoon potassium-chloride-based salt substitute, such as NoSalt
- ½ teaspoon white pepper

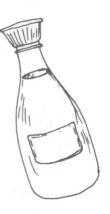

SOUP:

- 4 ounces brown rice noodles
- 1 quart low-sodium chicken broth

- ½–⅔ package coleslaw mix (shredded cabbage and carrots)
- ½ tablespoon reduced-sodium soy sauce
- Optional toppings: toasted sesame oil, chopped scallions, chopped cilantro, Asian chili sauce (sambal oelek), chili garlic sauce, white pepper

1. Turn on a small food processor with the cover in place and toss garlic cloves into blades, chopping until fine. Turn off processor, remove top, and toss in pork cubes. Replace top and process until pork is finely ground and blended with garlic. Remove lid and transfer meat and garlic to a 1-quart bowl.

2. Place the chopped green cabbage and scallion in the food processor and pulse until finely chopped. Add to bowl with pork mixture. Add ginger, reduced-sodium soy sauce, sherry, sesame oil, salt substitute, and white pepper. Blend with a fork until well combined. Cover the bowl and refrigerate for at least 30 minutes.

3. Cook brown rice noodles according to package directions. Drain, rinse, and leave in the colander.

4. Bring the broth to a boil over high heat in a 3-quart pot. Meanwhile, remove the pork mixture from the refrigerator and form into small meatballs, using wet hands and placing meatballs on a large plate.

5. Drop meatballs one at a time into simmering broth. Bring back to a simmer and cook for 4–5 minutes (small meatballs will cook quickly). Add the coleslaw mix to the soup, stir, bring back to a simmer, cover the pot, and cook over medium-low heat for 4–5 minutes. Add the soy sauce. Taste the broth and adjust seasoning, adding ½–1 teaspoon honey and/or 1 tablespoon dry sherry, if desired.

6. Rinse noodles with hot water to warm them up, and divide them between two large soup bowls. If desired, add a drizzle of toasted sesame oil to noodles. Pour the soup mixture and meatballs over noodles. Serve with optional toppings.

EASY MICROWAVE POLENTA

Makes 4 cups

Per cup—110 calories

Polenta is a traditional Northern Italian dish that is usually topped with flavorful stews and sauces. Made with whole grain cornmeal, it is an easy way to add whole grain to a meal. Traditional polenta is often made with cream or butter and cheese, but we have omitted them here to make it heart healthy. Polenta is also typically made by stirring over a hot stove for 20 to 30 minutes. Cooked in the microwave as directed here simplifies the process, yielding a smooth and comforting canvas for a saucy stew. Fine-ground cornmeal produces a silky, creamy texture, while coarse-ground cornmeal leads to a chewy, rough texture. Both are delicious. This recipe produces a soft, spoonable variety of polenta, akin to grits, rather than the harder, sliceable type that some recipes yield. Serve topped with an easy cacciatore made with chunks of chicken breast simmered in a healthy variety of jarred pasta sauce and a splash of red or white wine; add a sprinkling of grated Parmesan.

- 1 cup stone ground, whole grain yellow cornmeal (fine-ground or coarse-ground)
- 4 cups water
- ½ teaspoon salt substitute

1. Whisk all ingredients in a 3-quart microwave-safe bowl. Microwave, uncovered, for 5 minutes at 100% power (for 1,000–1,200-watt microwave oven).
2. Remove from the microwave, stir or whisk well to break up lumps, and return to the microwave, uncovered. Microwave at 100% power for 5 more minutes.
3. Remove from the microwave again, stir well again, and return to the microwave at 20% power for 10 minutes. Let stand in the microwave, or covered outside of the microwave, for 10 minutes before serving.
4. To serve, spoon into bowls or onto plates and top with a saucy entrée.

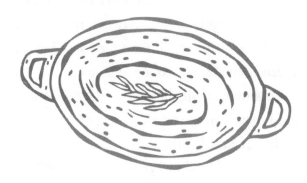

ITALIAN-STYLE SPAGHETTI SQUASH BAKE

Makes 4 servings

Per serving—322 calories

This is a fun way to use spaghetti squash. Blending the squash strands with Parmesan and other seasonings gives major flavor to this bland vegetable. Layering the squash with a simple tomato sauce and low-fat cheese makes a cozy, filling meal.

- 2½ pounds spaghetti squash
- ½ cup water
- ¼ cup grated Parmesan, divided
- ½ teaspoon potassium-chloride salt substitute, such as NoSalt
- 1 teaspoon black pepper
- 1 tablespoon olive oil
- 3 large garlic cloves, minced
- 1 medium onion, chopped
- ½ pound mushrooms, sliced
- 14.5-ounce can diced tomatoes, no salt added
- ½ teaspoon dried basil or 1 tablespoon fresh chopped basil
- ½ teaspoon crushed red pepper flakes
- 1 cup shredded part-skim mozzarella
- ⅔ cup part-skim or fat-free ricotta

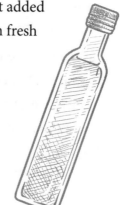

1. Cut the spaghetti squash in half. Remove seeds with a large spoon and discard. In a microwave-safe dish, place the squash halves cut side down and add ½ cup water. Microwave at full power, uncovered, until tender, about 12 minutes.

2. Remove the squash and use a fork to scrape squash into a 2-quart bowl. Discard the shells. To squash in the bowl, add 2 tablespoons Parmesan, ½ teaspoon black pepper, and ¼ teaspoon salt substitute. Mix well and cover to warm.

3. Heat the olive oil in a skillet or 2-quart sauce pan. Add the garlic, onions, and mushrooms, sautéing until softened. Add canned tomatoes, basil, ½ teaspoon black pepper, ¼ teaspoon salt substitute, and crushed red pepper flakes. Bring to a boil and simmer for 5 minutes.

4. Spray an 8 x 8-inch baking dish with olive oil cooking spray or brush with olive oil. Spread ⅓ of the squash mixture in the bottom of the dish, add ⅓ of the sauce, sprinkle with ⅓ cup mozzarella, and dollop with ⅓ cup ricotta. Repeat one more time with squash, sauce, mozzarella, and the rest of the ricotta. For the third time, use the final third of the squash mixture, the final third of the sauce, and the rest of the mozzarella. Sprinkle the remaining 2 tablespoons of Parmesan evenly over top of dish.

5. Bake at 375°F for 20–25 minutes, until cheese is bubbling. Remove from the oven and let cool for 5 minutes. Divide into 4 servings.

TACO LASAGNA

Makes 6 servings*

Per serving—308 calories

INGREDIENTS:

- ½ pound 93% lean ground turkey
- ½ packet (1.25 ounces) no-salt taco seasoning mix (such as Mrs. Dash, or make your own**)
- 2 garlic cloves, minced
- ¼–½ teaspoon cayenne pepper (to taste)
- ½ tablespoon chili powder
- ¼ cup water
- 9 (6-inch) yellow corn tortillas
- 1½ cups salsa (or ½ of 24-ounce jar) or 1½ cups homemade salsa***
- ½ cup sliced scallions
- 1 cup light sour cream or nonfat Greek yogurt
- ¾ cup (3 ounces) shredded low-fat cheddar
- ¾ cup (3 ounces) shredded part-skim mozzarella
- 2 tablespoons chopped cilantro (optional)

DIRECTIONS:

1. Brown ground turkey in a nonstick skillet until no longer pink. Add the taco seasoning, garlic, cayenne pepper, chili powder, and water. Simmer for 10 minutes.
2. Preheat oven to 375°F. Spray the bottom of a 8 x 8-inch baking dish with olive oil cooking spray.

3. Arrange 3 tortillas to cover the bottom of the prepared baking dish, cutting in half to fit. Spread ½ cup salsa on top. Spread half of the meat mixture evenly over the salsa. Dollop half of the sour cream randomly over the meat mixture. Sprinkle with ¼ cup sliced scallions. Top with ¼ cup cheddar and ¼ cup mozzarella.

4. Repeat layers, starting with 3 tortillas.

5. Top with remaining 3 tortillas, spread with remaining salsa, and sprinkle with remaining cheeses.

6. Bake in the preheated oven for 30–35 minutes, or until cheeses are melted.

7. To serve, cut into 6 rectangles. Sprinkle each serving with chopped cilantro.

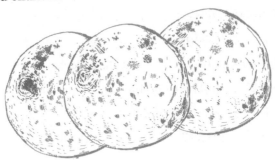

*If doubling the Taco Lasagna recipe for 12 servings, use a 9 x 13-inch baking dish. Bake 40–45 minutes.

**To make your own "packet" of low-sodium taco seasoning, combine 1 tablespoon chili powder, 1½ teaspoons ground cumin, ¼ teaspoon each onion powder, garlic powder, oregano, and crushed red pepper flakes, ½ teaspoon paprika, ½ teaspoon black pepper, and ½ teaspoon salt substitute, such as NoSalt. (The salt substitute is optional; you may find that this dish is flavorful enough without adding the salt substitute.) Use half of this mixture for the Taco Lasagna or the entire mixture if you double the recipe.

***Easy Homemade Salsa—Combine 1 medium or 2 small chopped tomatoes, with their juice, to make about 1½ cups (or one 14.5-ounce can diced, no-salt tomatoes, with ½ cup juice), ½ small chopped onion, and 1 sprig of chopped cilantro. Place in a bowl with 1 small clove of minced garlic. Add 1 small chopped jalapeno or other hot pepper, if desired. Season with a squeeze of lime juice, a splash of distilled vinegar, or ¼ teaspoon potassium-chloride salt substitute, such as NoSalt.

STROGANOFF CASSEROLE

Makes about 10 cups (if pasta is cooked until very soft)
Per cup—247 calories

This easy, healthier take on stroganoff ditches the butter and cream for olive oil and a touch of light sour cream, adding a little grated Parmesan to punch up the flavor. The red wine provides a delicious background note. Instead of egg noodles, this recipe uses whole wheat rotini. Serve with a salad.

- ½ pound whole wheat rotini
- 2 tablespoons olive oil
- 1 medium onion, finely chopped
- 3 garlic cloves, minced
- 8 ounces thickly sliced brown mushrooms, such as baby bella (crimini)
- 1 pound 93% lean ground turkey or ground bison
- 2 tablespoons flour
- Two 8-ounce cans no-salt tomato sauce
- ½ cup dry red wine
- 1½ cups no-salt beef broth
- 1–2 teaspoons potassium-chloride-based salt substitute, such as NoSalt
- 1 teaspoon black pepper
- ½ cup light sour cream
- ½ cup grated Parmesan

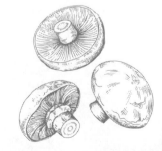

1. Bring 3 quarts water to a boil in a large pot. Add the rotini and cook, stirring occasionally, until very soft, 20–25 minutes. Turn off the heat and let the pasta sit in the hot water until ready to assemble the casserole. This longer cooking time expands the pasta and makes it silkier, more like the egg noodles the rotini is replacing.

2. Heat the olive oil in 3-quart pan. Add the onion, garlic, and mushrooms. Sauté over medium-high heat until softened, about 5 minutes. Add the ground turkey and sauté, stirring to break up the meat, until no longer pink.

3. Sprinkle flour over the meat mixture and stir well. Add the tomato sauce, red wine, broth, salt substitute, and black pepper. Bring to a boil, reduce heat to low, and simmer, uncovered, for 10 minutes, stirring occasionally. Turn off the heat and blend in the sour cream. Taste and adjust seasonings, adding ½–1 teaspoon honey if desired.

4. Drain the pasta in a colander. Spray a 3- or 4-quart casserole or oven-safe bowl with olive oil cooking spray, or lightly brush inside with olive oil. Spread one-quarter of the pasta in the bottom of casserole. Add one-quarter of the sauce mixture and sprinkle lightly with about 1 tablespoon of Parmesan. Repeat three more times, spreading the remainder of the sauce evenly over the top. Sprinkle evenly with remaining Parmesan.

5. Bake, uncovered, at 375°F for 25 minutes.

SMOKY FISH AND VEGGIE BOWL

Makes 1 serving

Per serving if made with a 3.75-ounce can of sardines in oil—422 calories

This is an easy way to include omega-3-rich fish in a quick solo lunch or dinner. White potatoes give this a big boost of potassium, but you can try sweet potatoes, which pair well with salmon, if you prefer. Tinned fish and the microwave make this dish a breeze to prepare.

- 1 medium potato (6 ounces) cut into ½-inch cubes
- 1 medium carrot, sliced or diced
- 1 stalk celery, sliced or diced
- 1 small (3–4 ounces) tin of fish, such as sardines or herring steaks, in oil or hot sauce, or 5-ounce can of salmon
- 1–2 teaspoons tomato paste (Use the kind from a tube for an easy trick!)
- A few shakes of onion powder
- 2 teaspoons balsamic vinegar
- ¼ teaspoon smoked paprika or ½ teaspoon liquid smoke

1. Place the potato cubes in a 1-quart microwave safe bowl (or 4-cup microwave-safe measuring

cup). Cover with a microwave-safe plate and microwave on high for 3 minutes.

2. Remove the bowl from the microwave and stir the potatoes. Top with the carrots and cover with the plate. Microwave on high for 2 minutes.

3. Stir, add the celery, and cook another 1–2 minutes, leaving the carrots and celery a bit crunchy.

4. Remove from the microwave. Stir in the tomato paste and about 1 tablespoon water. Mix well. Add the tin of fish, including any liquid or oil in the can. Add the onion powder, balsamic vinegar, and smoked paprika or liquid smoke. Stir well. Add more seasonings to taste.

INDIAN-STYLE EGG ROLL-UPS (VEGETARIAN)

Makes 1 serving (1 roll-up + all of the slaw)
Per serving, if made with whole eggs—409 calories
Per serving, if made with egg substitute—306 calories

This yummy, easy meal can be expanded to as many mouths as you have to feed! The tangy, slaw-like topping also makes a great side dish or salad. You can grate the vegetables quickly by using the grating blade on a food processor.

FOR EACH PERSON:

- 1 medium carrot, grated
- 1 small or ½ large cucumber, peeled, seeded, and grated
- ½ small onion, peeled and grated
- 1–2 tablespoons chopped cilantro
- 1–2 tablespoons low-salt, low-sugar ketchup
- ½—1 tablespoon rice vinegar or apple cider vinegar
- Black pepper, to taste
- Sriracha, to taste
- ½ teaspoon honey, if needed
- 2 high-omega-3 eggs or 6 tablespoons egg substitute
- 1–2 teaspoons olive oil
- 1 whole wheat tortilla, soft-taco-sized

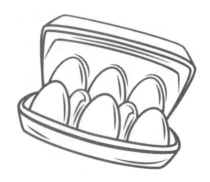

1. Combine the carrot, cucumber, onion, cilantro, ketchup, vinegar, black pepper, and sriracha in small bowl. Stir well and taste for seasoning. Add honey if too tangy. Set aside.

2. Heat a small, nonstick skillet over medium heat. Add the olive oil and heat until shimmering.

3. Meanwhile, beat 2 eggs well or measure out ½ cup egg substitute; add to the hot oil in the skillet. Let cook for 1–2 minutes, then place tortilla directly on top of the egg in the skillet. This will seal tortilla to egg. Allow to cook for about 2 minutes more, then lift a small section of the egg with a spatula to check for browning. Egg is done when it is golden brown underneath. Flip onto serving plate so that the egg portion is on top. If you are making more than one, cover each one with an inverted plate after cooking to keep warm.

4. Top egg and tortilla with some of the carrot-cucumber slaw. Roll up, if desired, and eat like a burrito, or serve open-faced with a knife and fork. (Open-faced presentation allows you to pile on more of the tangy slaw.) Serve remaining carrot-cucumber slaw on the side.

SOUTHWESTERN BEANS AND RICE (VEGETARIAN)

Makes 4 servings

Per serving without toppings—380 calories

This simple, one-pot, plant-based meal combines brown rice, black beans, and other heart-healthy ingredients with flavors of the southwest. It is surprisingly satisfying for low effort. This gets a "Yum!" from most diners!

- 1 tablespoon olive oil
- 1 cup long grain brown rice
- 1 large onion, chopped
- 2–3 garlic cloves, put through press
- 2 tablespoons chili powder
- ½ teaspoon cayenne pepper (optional)
- 2–3 teaspoons ground cumin
- ½–1 teaspoon potassium-chloride salt substitute, such as NoSalt
- ½–1 teaspoon black pepper
- 14.5-ounce can no-salt diced tomatoes with juice
- 1½ cups water
- 15-ounce can no-salt black beans, drained
- 1 cup drained, canned, no-salt corn or 1 cup frozen corn
- Toppings: chopped cilantro, salsa, low-fat shredded cheese, nonfat Greek yogurt

1. In 3-quart pan, heat the olive oil until shimmering and add the rice. Sauté until the rice is shiny and slightly brown. Toss in onion and garlic and sauté over medium heat until softened. Add the chili powder, cayenne pepper, cumin, salt substitute, and black pepper. Stir to combine well.

2. Add the tomatoes and water. Bring to a simmer, stir, cover, and reduce the heat to low to maintain a simmer. Cook for 30 minutes, until liquid is absorbed and rice is tender but not soggy. Stir to loosen up the rice.

3. Stir in the corn and beans. Cover and heat over low heat until warmed through. Turn off heat and allow to sit, undisturbed, for 10 minutes. Taste and adjust seasonings.

4. Serve with chopped cilantro and other toppings.

SLOW COOKER "ROAST" CHICKEN

Makes about 6 servings

Per serving, without optional gravy, if made with 3-pound chicken—312 calories

This chicken recipe is simple and flavorful. Removing the skin before cooking produces a lovely, low-fat chicken broth. The broth can be turned into a silky gravy or used in soups or to flavor potatoes, whole grain pasta, or farro. After slow cooking, the chicken is soft and mouth-wateringly juicy. Much like rotisserie chicken, the meat is great in salads, tucked into whole grain wraps, added to soups, eaten as is with veggies and a healthy starch, or used as the base for other recipes.

- 3–4-pound chicken
- ½ cup water
- 1–2 teaspoons onion powder

1. Place chicken, breast side up, in a clean kitchen sink. Remove any wrapping and remove neck and giblets if tucked into the cavity.

2. Using kitchen shears, make a vertical cut through the skin over the breast and peel back, removing all skin from breast and legs. Continue tugging at and removing the remainder of the skin from the chicken, using shears to cut off stubborn sections. Use shears to remove deposits of yellow or white fat on back, legs, and other areas. When you are done, most of the skin and fat should be gone.

3. Place the chicken, breast side up, in a slow cooker. An oval-shaped cooker provides the best fit. Pour in ½ cup water. Sprinkle chicken with onion powder.

4. Set cooker to low and cook 3–5 hours, depending on your slow cooker. Check for doneness by inserting a meat thermometer into the breast. Chicken is done when the thermometer registers 165°F.

5. Using two large cooking spoons, transfer the chicken to a large bowl or platter. Carve the chicken into pieces or pull meat into shreds or chunks and discard the bones.

6. The chicken broth can be thickened for gravy by turning the slow cooker to high heat, making sure that the broth is very hot, and adding a slurry of cornstarch and water. Start with 2 tablespoons cornstarch mixed with 2 tablespoons water and add to hot broth, stirring until thickened. If not thick enough, add more cornstarch and water. Season with pepper, onion powder, and salt substitute, if desired.

QUICK CHICKEN CURRY

Makes 4 servings
Per serving, if made with chicken breast, without rice—350 calories
Per serving, if made with chicken thighs, without rice—365 calories
With rice—add 108 calories per ½ cup cooked brown rice

Cooking this dish is an easy way to fill your house with the delicious smell of curry. Green beans make a great side dish.

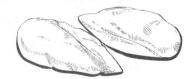

- 1½ pounds boneless, skinless chicken pieces (breasts or thighs)
- 1 cup no-salt chicken broth
- 2 tablespoons cornstarch
- ¾ cup nonfat evaporated milk (or ½ cup light coconut milk + ¼ cup water)
- 1 small onion, chopped, or 2 tablespoons dried minced onion
- 1 teaspoon salt substitute (optional)
- 1 tablespoon curry powder
- 1 teaspoon honey
- 1 teaspoon onion powder
- ½ teaspoon garlic powder
- 4-ounce can unsalted mushrooms, drained
- ¼ cup raisins
- ¼ cup unsalted roasted peanuts
- Cooked brown rice, for serving

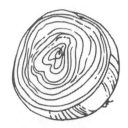

1. Cut the chicken into strips or chunks. Arrange chicken in the bottom of a 3-quart microwave-safe casserole with cover.

2. Combine chicken broth and cornstarch in a 1-quart microwave-safe bowl or a 1-quart measuring cup. Microwave on high for 1 minute. Stir and microwave again for 30 seconds. Stir again and add evaporated milk (or coconut milk and water), onion, and seasonings and blend well. Add the rest of the ingredients and stir.

3. Pour broth and seasoning mixture over chicken. Cover the casserole.

4. Microwave on high (100% power) for 8 minutes (1,000–1,200-watt microwave). Stir. If chicken is not done (165°F), replace cover and cook at 50% power for 5 more minutes. Let stand 5 minutes to complete cooking. Remove from microwave and check the chicken for doneness.

5. Serve over brown rice. Top with more peanuts and raisins, if desired.

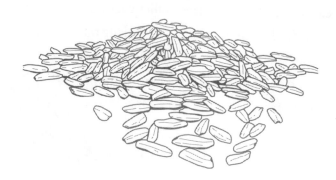

CRUSTLESS SPINACH QUICHE

Makes 8 servings
Per serving, if made with whole eggs—171 calories
Per serving, if made with egg substitute—143 calories

This easy quiche is great served with steamed, baked, or roasted potatoes. Omitting the crust saves time and removes the saturated fat found in most pie crusts.

- 1 tablespoon olive oil
- 1 medium onion, chopped
- 10-ounce package frozen spinach, chopped or whole leaf, thawed
- 5 high-omega-3 whole eggs or 1¼ cups egg substitute
- ½ cup skim milk
- 8 ounces (2 cups) shredded low-fat sharp cheddar cheese
- ⅛ teaspoon black pepper

1. Preheat oven to 350°F. Spray a 9-inch pie pan or Pyrex pie dish with olive oil cooking spray.
2. Heat the olive oil in a large skillet over medium-high heat. Add the onions and cook, stirring occasionally, until the onions are soft. Stir in the spinach and continue cooking until excess moisture has evaporated.

3. In a large bowl, combine eggs, milk, cheese, and pepper. Add spinach mixture and stir to blend. Scoop into prepared pie pan.

4. Bake in preheated oven until eggs have set, about 30 minutes. Let cool for 10 minutes before serving. Cut into 8 wedges.

MICROWAVE EGGPLANT PARMIGIANA

Makes 4 generous servings

Per serving, if made with low-fat, low-sodium marinara sauce—289 calories

Per serving, if made with regular jarred marinara sauce—330 calories

Here's a quick version of eggplant parmigiana. Serve with a crisp salad. Leaving the skin on the eggplant retains the anthocyanins, which are antioxidants that reduce the risk of heart disease.

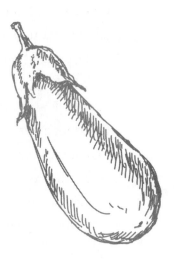

- 1 large eggplant (1½–2 pound)
- 3 slices whole wheat bread, toasted
- 2 tablespoons extra virgin olive oil
- 1 teaspoon onion powder
- 3 tablespoons grated Parmesan cheese
- 1 cup (4 ounces) shredded low-fat mozzarella cheese
- 1¾ cups low-sodium marinara sauce

1. Slice eggplant into ½-inch slices. Arrange slices in a large, microwave-safe bowl. Microwave for 3 minutes on high. Remove from the microwave and let cool. Drain any liquid that has collected in the bowl.

2. Meanwhile, tear toasted bread into small pieces. Place in a food processor and process into crumbs. Drizzle the olive oil and onion powder into the bread crumbs and process until well combined.

3. Spray a 9-inch square baking dish or a 2-quart covered casserole with olive oil cooking spray. Spread about ¼ cup pasta sauce into the bottom of the dish. Arrange one-third of the drained eggplant slices over the sauce. Sprinkle with one-third of the bread crumb mixture. Drizzle ½ cup marinara sauce over bread crumbs. Sprinkle with 1 tablespoon Parmesan cheese and ⅓ cup mozzarella. Repeat two more layers, ending with mozzarella.

4. Cover the dish with a microwave-safe plate or cover if using a casserole. Microwave on medium (50% power) for 10 minutes. Check for doneness (microwave ovens vary); eggplant should be soft and cheese should be bubbling. Check the temperature at the center of the casserole with an instant-read thermometer, if you have one. The center should register 165°F. If not hot enough, cover and cook on medium for another 5 minutes.

5. Let stand 5 minutes before cutting into 4 servings.

ASIAN PORK TENDERLOIN

Makes 4 servings

Per serving—215 calories

This dish stars pork tenderloin, the leanest cut of red meat. The flavorful marinade adds an Asian touch to this tender meat. Take care not to overcook—pork tenderloin is safe to eat at an internal temp of 145°F, when it will still be juicy. It may be a pale pink inside. (In 2020, the USDA revised their recommended cooking temperatures for meats. https://www.usda.gov/media/blog/2011/05/25/cooking-meat-check-new-recommended-temperatures) Serve with brown rice and steamed or stir-fried bok choy, broccoli, or other leafy green.

- 2 tablespoons reduced-sodium soy sauce
- 2 tablespoons honey
- 2 tablespoons dry sherry
- 1 tablespoon canola oil or non-extra-virgin olive oil
- ½ teaspoon garlic powder
- ½ teaspoon cinnamon
- 1 pound pork tenderloin, trimmed of fat

1. Combine the reduced-sodium soy sauce, honey, sherry, oil, garlic powder, and cinnamon in a shallow baking dish large enough to accommodate the pork tenderloin. Mix well.

2. Add the pork tenderloin to the dish and roll around to coat with marinade. Cover and marinate in the refrigerator for at least 3 hours, turning occasionally to distribute marinade over meat.

3. Remove pork from the dish and save the marinade to use for basting the meat.

4. Place pork on preheated grill or grill pan.

   a. If using a grill, grill for 5 minutes per side, then check internal temperature with an instant-read thermometer. If less than 145°F, continue cooking for about 5 more minutes per side, checking temperature until 145°F is reached. Remove from grill.

   b. If using a grill pan, preheat oven to 425°F. Preheat grill pan over high heat. Add pork and sear on both sides, then continue to cook for 5 minutes per side. Place pork in shallow, oven-proof dish and bake for 10–15 minutes, checking internal temperature with an instant-read thermometer. Remove from oven when pork reaches 145°F and place pork on cutting board or platter.

5. Let pork rest for 3–5 minutes before cutting into ½-inch slices.

SLOW COOKER SPANISH RICE

Makes about 9 cups with riced cauliflower (6 cups without riced cauliflower)
Per 1½ cups, if made with riced cauliflower—303 calories
Per 1½ cups, if made without the riced cauliflower—445 calories

Combining brown rice and riced cauliflower provides a lighter texture to this slow cooker meal. Leave out the riced cauliflower, if you wish—the recipe will then yield about 6 cups. Serve with a crisp green salad.

- 1 pound 93% lean ground turkey
- 1 large red pepper
- 1 large onion
- 1 garlic clove
- 28-ounce can no-salt diced tomatoes
- 8-ounce can no-salt tomato sauce
- 1 cup brown rice
- ½ 12-ounce package frozen riced cauliflower, thawed
- 1 cup water
- 2 teaspoons potassium-based salt substitute
- 1 tablespoon chili powder
- 1 teaspoon smoked paprika
- ½ teaspoon garlic powder
- 2 packets sodium-free beef flavor granulated bouillon
- 2 tablespoons chopped cilantro stems (optional)
- 1 teaspoon cayenne pepper (optional)

1. Sauté ground turkey in a large skillet until browned. Pour into a slow cooker.

2. In a food processor, combine red pepper, onion, and garlic. Puree until mostly smooth. Add to slow cooker.

3. Add tomatoes, tomato sauce, brown rice, riced cauliflower, water, and all seasonings to slow cooker. Stir well.

4. Cover and cook for 5 hours on low and 3 hours on high, or until rice is tender. Adjust seasonings to taste.

VEGETARIAN WEST AFRICAN STEW (GROUNDNUT STEW)

Makes 6 servings

Per serving—341 calories

This easy, slow-cooker meal combines soluble-fiber–rich sweet potatoes and red beans with the heart-healthy goodness of onion, garlic, ginger, tomatoes, and peanuts. In West Africa, peanuts are called groundnuts because they grow underground. While the ingredient list for this recipe may look formidable, many of these items are common pantry staples. This stew is often made with chicken, but here we opt for a plant-based version.

- 1 tablespoon olive oil
- 1 large onion, chopped
- 2 garlic cloves, crushed
- 1½ pounds (2 medium) sweet potatoes, peeled, cut into ½-inch cubes

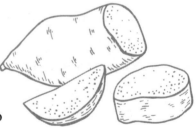

- 15-ounce can small red beans, drained and rinsed
- 1 cup reduced-sodium vegetable broth
- 1 medium red bell pepper, chopped
- 2 teaspoons grated fresh ginger
- ½ teaspoon cumin and/or ½ teaspoon ground coriander
- ½ teaspoon black pepper
- ½ teaspoon cayenne pepper (optional)

- Two 10-ounce cans diced tomatoes with green chilies
- ¼ cup natural creamy peanut butter
- ¼ cup chopped unsalted roasted peanuts
- Lime wedges

1. Sauté onion and garlic in the olive oil until softened. Place in a large slow cooker.
2. Add sweet potatoes, beans, broth, bell pepper, seasonings, and tomatoes to the slow cooker.
3. Cook on low until vegetables are softened, about 4 hours.
4. Ladle 1 cup cooking liquid into a measuring cup. Whisk in peanut butter. Add mixture to crock pot and stir. Cover and let flavors blend for 5–10 minutes. Adjust seasoning with more peanut butter, cayenne, coriander, cumin, or black pepper to taste.
5. Serve in bowls, topped with chopped peanuts and a squeeze of lime juice.

BLACK BEAN QUINOA SALAD

Makes about 8 servings as a side dish, 4 servings as an entrée
Per cup (side dish)—238 calories

Quinoa is a high-protein grain filled with soluble fiber. Finding tasty ways to serve it can be a challenge. This dish combines quinoa with fiber-filled, high-protein black beans and bright flavors to please most palates. Also, here's a tip: while many recipes call for rinsing the quinoa before cooking, most quinoa sold in the United States is already rinsed (check the bag's label). So usually, no rinsing is necessary.

- 1 cup quinoa
- 2 cups water
- 3 tablespoons sherry vinegar
- 1 tablespoon reduced-sodium soy sauce
- 1 tablespoon lime juice
- 1 canned chipotle pepper in adobo, minced (or ½ teaspoon smoked paprika)
- 4 tablespoons extra virgin olive oil
- 1 bunch scallions, sliced thinly
- 1 small red or white onion, finely chopped
- 1 red, yellow, or orange bell pepper, finely chopped
- 2–3 sprigs cilantro, chopped (or more to taste)
- Two 15-ounce cans low-sodium black beans, drained and rinsed

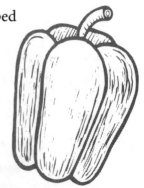

1. In a medium saucepan, combine the water and quinoa. Bring to a boil, cover, and cook on low for about 15 minutes, or until water has been absorbed. Remove from heat and allow to cool.

2. In a serving bowl, combine the sherry vinegar, reduced-sodium soy sauce, lime juice, chipotle, and extra virgin olive oil and whisk until well combined. Add the quinoa, black beans, and the rest of the ingredients and toss gently or stir to combine well.

3. Allow flavors to blend at room temperature for an hour, or refrigerate overnight until ready to serve. If refrigerated, let come to room temperature before serving.

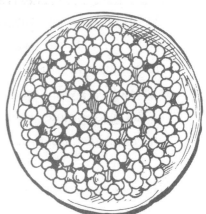

BEET BROWNIES

Makes 16 servings

Per serving (2-inch square)—141 calories

Beets are full of heart-healthy nitrates and phytochemicals, but they are not everyone's favorite vegetable. What could be better than burying this earthy vegetable in a pan of brownies? The surprising result accentuates the sweet notes of beets, tempering the bitterness of the cocoa powder. Cocoa and dark chocolate add to the heart-healthy qualities of this fun dessert. It is definitely worth a try! Experiment with baking times for your oven—you can make them fudgier by undercooking or cakier by using the full baking time. They become even fudgier if refrigerated and eaten the next day!

- 1 cup unsweetened dark cocoa powder (Dutch processed)
- 1 teaspoon baking soda
- ⅔ cup no-salt sliced beets from can or jar, drained and cut into chunks
- ½ cup dark brown sugar
- 2 teaspoons vanilla extract
- 7 ounces (about 1 cup) dark chocolate chips
- 2 tablespoons non-extra-virgin olive oil
- 2 large high-omega-3 eggs or 4 egg whites

1. Lightly grease an 8 x 8-inch baking pan with olive oil or spray with olive oil cooking spray.

2. Combine the cocoa powder and baking soda in a small bowl, whisking until fully combined.

3. Combine the sliced beets, brown sugar, and vanilla extract in a food processor. Process until pureed but not fully smooth. You may need to scrape down the sides of the processor bowl and pulse again.

4. Preheat oven to 350°F.

5. In a 2-cup microwave-safe measuring cup, combine ¾ cup chocolate chips and 2 tablespoons olive oil. Melt chips in a microwave in 15–20-second intervals, stirring each time, until chocolate is mostly melted. Remove from microwave and stir until completely smooth.

6. Add melted chocolate to the food processor with the beets. Puree with the beets until blended.

7. Add the eggs or egg whites and blend again. Scrape down the sides of the bowl.

8. Add the dry ingredients to the mixture in the food processor and puree just until well blended, scraping down the sides of the bowl to incorporate all ingredients. The batter will be very thick and fudgy.

9. Remove the bowl from the food processor, remove the blade, and carefully scrape batter from the blade and bowl into a prepared pan. Using your hands or a spatula,

push batter down and flatten across the pan to an even thickness. This will ensure uniform baking.

10. Scatter the remaining ounce of chocolate chips across the batter, spreading out evenly. Bake in preheated oven for 25–30 minutes. Brownies will be puffy on the edges and fudgier in the center when poked with a toothpick.

11. Place on a wire rack to cool. Let cool for 30 minutes or more before cutting into sixteen 2-inch squares. Can be refrigerated after cooling, which adds to their fudgy quality!

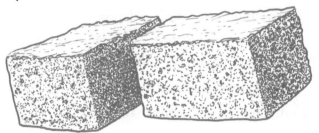

PATATAS BRAVAS (SPICY SPANISH POTATOES)

Makes 6 servings

Per serving—280 calories

This smoky, spicy potato dish (translated "fierce potatoes" for their spiciness) is a popular tapa in Spain, served with wine. These potatoes are also a nice complement to grilled salmon or chicken breast or an omelet made with high-omega-3 eggs or egg whites.

POTATOES:

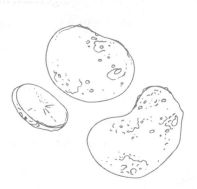

- 2 pounds red-skinned or Yukon Gold potatoes with skin, cut into 1-inch chunks
- ¼ cup extra virgin olive oil
- 1 teaspoon garlic powder

SALSA BRAVA:

- 2 tablespoons extra virgin olive oil
- 1 small onion, finely chopped
- 3 garlic cloves, crushed
- 28-ounce can no-salt crushed tomatoes
- 1½ teaspoons smoked paprika
- ½ teaspoon cayenne pepper
- ¼–½ teaspoon potassium-based salt substitute (optional)
- Hot sauce (optional)

FOR POTATOES:

1. Preheat oven to 450°F. In a medium bowl, coat the potato pieces with ¼ cup olive oil and garlic powder. Spread on a baking sheet.

2. Bake for 20–25 minutes, stirring once or twice, until tender and crispy.

FOR SALSA BRAVA:

3. While potatoes are roasting, in a large skillet, sauté the onion in 2 tablespoons olive oil until golden. Add garlic and cook, stirring, until well incorporated into the onion.

4. Add tomatoes and all seasonings, stir well, and bring to a simmer.

5. Simmer, uncovered, for 20 minutes, stirring occasionally. Taste and adjust seasonings.

6. Remove from heat and allow to cool.

7. Once cooled, the sauce can be pureed in a food processor. However, if you like the chunky texture, serve as is.

PRESENTATION:

8. Divide potatoes among shallow bowls.

9. Top with salsa brava.

TOFU PARMIGIANA

Makes 4 servings

Per serving—286 calories

Tofu can be a polarizing ingredient, but not in this dish. The familiar flavors of tomato and cheese, along with the pleasing texture of sliced baby bella mushrooms, give this riff on chicken parmigiana a homey feel. Brown mushrooms provide a higher level of the antioxidant ergothioneine than white mushrooms; studies on ergothioneine show its promise in supporting cardiometabolic health. This dish comes together in one skillet—without the oven! Serve with whole wheat or whole grain pasta and a green salad.

- 14-ounce package extra-firm tofu, drained
- ¼ teaspoon garlic powder
- ¼ cup whole wheat bread crumbs (1 slice whole wheat bread, toasted, crumbed in food processor)
- 1 teaspoon dried parsley flakes
- ¼ teaspoon dried oregano
- ¼ teaspoon dried basil
- 5 teaspoons olive oil
- 1 small onion, chopped
- ½ pound sliced baby bella (crimini) mushrooms
- ¼ cup grated Parmesan
- ¾ cup low-sodium marinara sauce
- ½ cup shredded part-skim mozzarella

1. Cut tofu into 4 long slices. Sprinkle with garlic powder on both sides.
2. Combine the bread crumbs, parsley flakes, dried oregano, and dried basil in a wide, shallow bowl or 8 x 8-inch dish.
3. Dredge tofu slices in bread crumb mixture.
4. In a large nonstick skillet over medium, heat 2 teaspoons olive oil. Sauté onion until brown. Add mushrooms and cook until moisture has evaporated and mushrooms begin to crisp. Transfer to a bowl.
5. Warm remaining 3 teaspoons olive oil in the same skillet. Add all four breaded tofu slices to the pan and cook until brown on first side, then flip over. Sprinkle each slice with 1 tablespoon Parmesan.
6. Top slices of tofu with mushroom mixture, then pour 3 tablespoons marinara sauce and 2 tablespoons mozzarella over each tofu slice. Cover and cook until cheese has melted, 3–5 minutes.

BEET HUMMUS

Makes 1 ½ cups

Per 2 tablespoons—63 calories

Here's another way to use heart-healthy beets, combined in a tasty hummus with other heart-healthy ingredients. Serve with sliced raw vegetables and whole grain, low-salt crackers.

- 1 cup no-salt sliced beets, drained
- 2 garlic cloves, pressed through garlic press
- 15-ounce can chickpeas, drained (reserve liquid for aquafaba recipes)
- 2 tablespoons tahini
- 2 tablespoons extra virgin olive oil
- 2–3 tablespoons lemon juice
- 2–3 tablespoons warm water
- ½ teaspoon cumin and/or coriander (optional)
- Freshly ground black pepper (optional)

1. Place beets in the bowl of a food processor. Process until chunky.
2. Add garlic, chickpeas, tahini, and olive oil and process until smooth. Add lemon juice and warm water, a little at a time, adjusting for desired texture and brightness. Taste and add remaining seasonings, if desired. Blend until combined. Adjust seasonings to taste.
3. Chill to blend flavors before serving.

BLACK BEAN DIP AND SPREAD

Makes 8 servings (2 cups)

Per ¼ cup—82 calories

Use this delicious dip as a meal starter for a gathering or as a light meal if you are too tired to cook. Also delicious as a sandwich filling when spread on toasted whole grain bread or stuffed into a warm whole wheat pita with shredded veggies. Besides being tasty, the black beans, garlic, and spices offer many heart-healthy properties.

- 15-ounce can no-salt black beans, drained (reserve liquid to adjust thickness of spread) and rinsed (Save any unused liquid for aquafaba recipes.)
- 3 tablespoons salsa, fresh or jarred, of desired level of heat
- 2 scallions, chopped
- 2 garlic cloves, pressed through garlic press
- ½ cup fat-free Greek yogurt
- 1 teaspoon hot sauce, or to taste
- 2 teaspoons ground cumin
- 1 teaspoon ground coriander
- Optional toppings: black pepper, lime juice, chopped cilantro

1. Combine all ingredients in a food processor or blender. Process until smooth, adding reserved bean liquid to adjust texture.
2. Taste and adjust seasonings. Black pepper and lime juice can be added to taste. Sprinkle with cilantro before serving, if desired.
3. Serve with homemade baked corn tortilla chips (below) and raw veggies or as a tasty sandwich filling or spread.

BAKED CORN TORTILLA CHIPS

(About 8 calories per chip)

Stack a few whole grain corn tortillas and cut into "pizza-slice" triangles, 8 per tortilla. Spread out evenly on cookie sheet. Bake at 350°F until crispy, flipping and rearranging on baking sheet once while baking to avoid scorching. Watch carefully to prevent burning. Allow to cool briefly before serving.

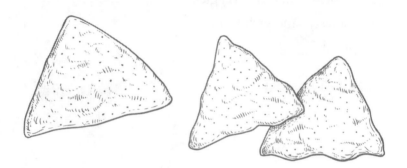

MEASUREMENT CONVERSIONS

Volume Equivalents (Liquid)

US Standard	US Standard (ounces)	Metric (approximate)
2 tablespoons	1 fl. oz.	20 mL
1/4 cup	2 fl. oz.	60 mL
1/2 cup	4 fl. oz.	120 mL
1 cup	8 fl. oz.	240 mL
1 1/2 cups	12 fl. oz.	355 mL
2 cups or 1 pint	16 fl. oz.	475 mL
4 cups or 1 quart	32 fl. oz.	1 L
1 gallon	128 fl. oz.	4 L

Volume Equivalents (Dry)

US Standard	Metric (approximate)
1/8 teaspoon	0.5 mL
1/4 teaspoon	1 mL
1/2 teaspoon	2 mL
3/4 teaspoon	4 mL
1 teaspoon	5 mL
1 tablespoon	15 mL
1/4 cup	59 mL
1/3 cup	79 mL
1/2 cup	118 mL
2/3 cup	156 mL
3/4 cup	177 mL
1 cup	235 mL
2 cups or 1 pint	475 mL
3 cups	700 mL
4 cups or 1 quart	1 L

Weight Equivalents

US Standard	Metric (approximate)
1/2 ounce	15 g
1 ounce	30 g
2 ounces	60 g
4 ounces	115 g
8 ounces	225 g
12 ounces	340 g
16 ounces or 1 pound	455 g

Oven Temperatures

Fahrenheit	Celsius (approximate)
250°F	120°C
300°F	150°C
325°F	165°C
350°F	180°C
375°F	190°C
400°F	200°C
425°F	220°C
450°F	230°C

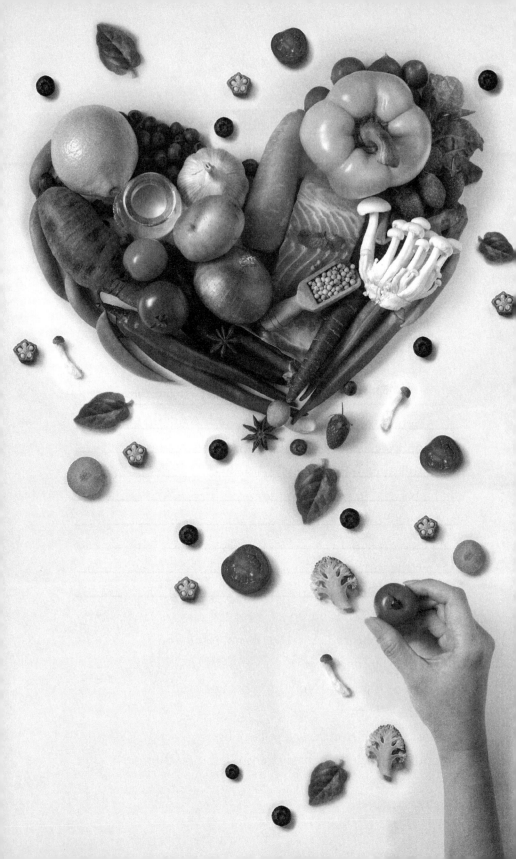

CHAPTER 8

Dr. Crandall's Simple Fitness Plan

Our body is built for action, so it's no wonder that lounging on the couch or sitting in front of the computer all day can result in your becoming overweight.

The best thing people can do for their hearts, regardless of age, is to follow a program of daily, moderate exercise.

As I have noted, I face my own battle with heart disease, and I know the difference that keeping fit makes in my own life. But even if I didn't have research or my patients to turn to, all I would need to do is observe history to know the best method for preventing heart disease. You might recall from my previous books that I'm an old anthropology student, so I know that although heart disease is our most common killer today, it used to be rare.

Consider prehistoric man: he spent his days walking in search of food. But society evolved over millennia, and heart disease became more common—but only for the upper class because they had the luxury of being sedentary.

Then the Industrial Revolution changed life for everyone. Machines took the place of manual labor, and we took to traveling in cars, trains, and planes. And it's even worse in the computer age. We no longer even have to walk to the mailbox; we just zip off an email.

Every little reason that we've had for keeping active has vanished, and we are paying for it with our health.

Because we no longer engage in active lives out of necessity, we must find ways to build physical activity into our daily routines to keep our hearts in good working order. That's why I've created "Dr. Crandall's Three-Point Plan to Keep Your Heart Young." It contains everything you need to know to get yourself active and keep your heart healthy.

Here's my plan in a nutshell:

- Walk Heart Disease Away
- Build and Retain Muscle Mass
- Activity Trumps Stress

Step 1. Walk Heart Disease Away

I walk for a full hour every day. I know this sounds simple, but don't fool yourself: Walking for 60 minutes each day requires commitment. But the benefits you reap will change your life.

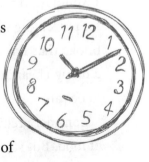

Walking is an aerobic exercise, which means your heartbeat is raised for a sustained period of time. You may have heard that 30 minutes, a few times per week, is sufficient to keep you healthy. I disagree. In fact, the reason those experts limit their recommendations to 30 minutes a few times per week is because they don't think people will have the discipline to walk for a full hour every day. I have more faith.

Still, an hour per day can seem like a daunting task. I usually tell my patients to start with 20 minutes each day for two weeks, then advance to 40 minutes each day for another two weeks. After a month of warming up, they are ready to make the commitment to walking a full hour every day.

What happens when you walk for an hour?

Do you remember when you were young, and as you kept running, you got that exhilarating "second wind" feeling? Well, that's not all in your head. It's actually your body adjusting once it has gone through its built-in energy reserve. And the results are remarkable.

We're all familiar with the body's circulatory system, which consists of the vessels and muscles that control the blood flow throughout the body. The components of this system include the heart, arteries, veins, and capillaries.

What you may not know is that your body also has what's called a "collateral circulatory system," a microscopic network of blood vessels that ordinarily remain closed. However, with sustained physical activity—such as a daily, hour-long walk—these vessels open and become enlarged, forming an alternate network to bring blood to your heart. When these vessels open, it causes the "second wind" feeling of prolonged, aerobic exercise.

In addition, this blood flow can detour around blockages and relieve angina (chest pain that comes from heart disease) or even help to prevent a heart attack.

But that's not all that one-hour walk does. As you continue beyond the 30-minute mark, your body pumps up its production of nitric oxide, a gas that is credited with many benefits, such as helping keep arteries clean of plaque as well as widening the arteries and keeping them supple. Each of these actions helps lower blood pressure, decreasing the risk of both heart attack and stroke.

Walking Is Just the Beginning

Want to add variety to your exercise plan? Swimming is great, of course, but even if you don't swim, don't overlook the water. Check with health clubs or local pools for water aerobics classes.

When I get home from work, I make sure to add an additional activity period to the day as well. So, after dinner, this means I hop on my stationary bike, or perhaps I take a swim, or even take another walk. The idea is to keep moving.

Before you start any physical activity program, consult your physician. Most people can manage a short walk and build up from there, unless they have serious health problems. But it's always best to be safe.

Step 2. Build and Retain Muscle Mass

Although sustained aerobic activity is the cornerstone of my plan—because it builds up your cardiovascular system, which leads to endurance, lower blood pressure, and better heart health—this is not the only type of exercise your body craves. For optimal health, you need to build muscle mass.

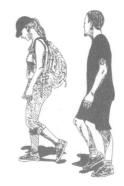

Once we pass age 50, our sex hormone levels drop (testosterone in men, estrogen in women), which causes muscle mass to diminish. When this happens, muscle is replaced with fat, and the flabby result shows in the mirror.

Regular strength training (also called resistance training) builds muscle and decreases the losses that are normally experienced with aging. Muscle tissue is very active and has high-energy requirements. This means that the more muscle you have (compared to fat), the more calories you can consume without gaining weight.

And there also are practical advantages to having more muscle mass. Added muscle tissue helps maintain strength and bolster endurance. Muscle allows you to do the things you love to do, such as bowling, gardening, or even playing with the grandkids.

Resistance training also combats frailty, which is a major factor in aging. This is true for both men and women, but it is in females that such training has been underemphasized. This is wrong—as a recent University of Buffalo study found.

Frailty is the condition of old age that results in weakness, fatigue, weight loss, and an inability to walk fast or exercise vigorously. People who are frail are often unable to keep up with the tasks of daily lives, and are more likely to end up in nursing homes.

This condition is too often thought of as an inevitable part of old age—but it is not. People who engage in building muscle mass can build strength at any age, studies find. Also, the muscle mass built up when you're younger—even in your 60s—can pay off when you are in your 70s, 80s, and even 90s.

Researchers looked at 46 women across two different age groups, 60–74 and 75–90. They found that, while frailty is progressive, those who built up strength at the younger age carried over this benefit and remained more mobile, even at advanced age, according to the study, published in *Physical and Occupational Therapy in Geriatrics*.

That's why it is so important to build strength training into your daily schedule.

Keep it interesting. When I first present my physical activity recommendations to my patients, they are generally very agreeable. As I said, they've often just had a heart attack and are scared, so they'll agree to anything.

But time passes, and their attitude changes. After all, we all lead busy lives, and finding the time to exercise on a daily basis is difficult.

But this is your *life* we are talking about. Start off the day with that walk, or write your time at the gym into your appointment book. Discipline yourself to build this type of activity into your day, every day. Remember, heart disease is progressive; it never stops. So you cannot stop, either. You need to stay active to beat it.

Here, then, are some ways to keep your activity program interesting:

Build in variety. Find a local walking track or bike trail, or drive to a park or a different neighborhood to explore a different environment. Keep it interesting.

Vary your program according to the season. You need to find a way to exercise year-round, whether you do so at home, at the gym, outdoors in good weather, or at a mall if it's rainy. (No pausing or window-shopping!)

Walk with your spouse or a friend. But make sure you're both committed to walking because chatting will slow you down. This is true, also, of walking with your dog. Save that type of walking for the additional activity because you won't reap all of the benefits of your hour-long walk.

Give ballroom dancing a whirl. Some of my oldest, happiest, and healthiest patients are ballroom dancers; they relish both the activity and the sociability that comes along with it. In many classes you don't need to come with a partner; the instructor will pair you up.

Step 3. Activity Trumps Stress

Stress is the body's response to an imminent threat. Once again, we can think back to our prehistoric ancestors to understand just how this process works.

Imagine a prehistoric man out in the open, searching for food, when a saber-toothed tiger suddenly comes across his path. His body had to spring into action to avoid becoming food himself.

Automatically, his adrenal glands started emitting hormones, including adrenalin and cortisol, to quicken his heart and get blood pumping to his legs to enable him to escape. This is what's known as the "fight-or-flight" response.

Although we aren't likely to encounter any saber-toothed tigers as we go about our daily life nowadays, we do get into stressful situations, such as fights with our bosses or financial troubles. In those cases, our adrenal glands keep churning out hormones. As a result, these hormones, particularly cortisol, remain in our bloodstream too long.

Cortisol is a toxic hormone, which can result in inflammation as well as the accumulation of pounds in the abdomen.

Fortunately, you can blunt the "flight-or-fight" response by being active. When you exercise, your body produces endorphins, which are hormones that act as natural mood elevators. This is how activity alleviates depression. Over time, the natural suppression of cortisol also will cause a drop in blood pressure.

By sticking to this three-step plan, you can reap the benefits of activity, which not only can forestall heart disease but also will have you feeling healthier than you have in years.

DR. CRANDALL'S MOTIVATIONAL TIP

Five Important Fitness Facts

1. Adding physical activity into your daily schedule is key to beating heart disease.
2. Building up to 10,000 steps is an excellent way to create a life-long exercise program.
3. You need at least three weekly periods of strength training to maintain your strength, even into old age.
4. If you pick activities you find fun and interesting, exercise won't seem like a chore.
5. Exercising with a friend or partner can add to your enjoyment of exercise.

ACKNOWLEDGMENTS

I would like to thank Newsmax CEO Christopher Ruddy for his belief and trust in my work; Mary Glenn, the publisher, and her team at Humanix; and my gifted and amazing co-author, Charlotte Libov.

I also want to acknowledge registered dietician and cooking enthusiast Sue Gebo for the recipes she contributed to this book.

INDEX

Y

ABOUT THE AUTHORS

Chauncey W. Crandall IV, M.D., F.A.C.C., is a renowned cardiologist in the United States and the leader of medical missions across the world for forty years, leading medical teams on the front lines of battle and waging a war against the plagues that devastate poor communities throughout the world.

He is Director of Preventive Medicine and Complex Cardiology at Palm Beach Cardiovascular Clinic in Palm Beach, Florida.

His passion for heading to medical crises all over the world began early, when, at the age of nineteen, he traveled to the jungles of Africa and worked stateside with world-famous anthropologist Colin M. Turnbull. He gained early training in pandemics at Yale University, where he was introduced to Dr. Robert Gallo, the virologist who discovered the HIV virus that can lead to AIDS. Over his career, Dr. Crandall has performed more than forty thousand heart procedures. He regularly lectures nationally and internationally on a variety of cardiology topics, and he is the author of several top-selling health books, including *The Simple Heart Cure*, and *Fight Back: Beat the Coronavirus*, and he is the editor of the popular medical newsletter *Dr. Crandall's Heart Health Report*.

Dr. Crandall continues to devote much of his life's work to the poor, the suffering, and the dying and personally ministers to the sick in areas forgotten by others.

He has been heralded for his values and message of hope and victory that he brings to his patients in the United States and that he spreads to others throughout the world.

To contact Dr. Crandall:

Dr. Chauncey Crandall

c/o Chadwick Foundation

P.O. Box 3046

Palm Beach, FL 33480

chaunceycrandall.com

Charlotte Libov is an award-winning author and speaker. Her first book, *The Women's Heart Book*, was one of the first to sound the alarm about heart disease in women being overlooked, and resulted in her becoming a well-known speaker and patient advocate, work she continues today. She is the author, co-author, or writer of several books, including *The Cancer Survival Guide* (American Society of Journalists and Authors' Self Help Book of the Year), *A Women's Guide to Heart Attack Recovery*, and *Beat Your Risk Factors*, and, most recently, *The Liver Cure*. She is a former *New York Times* contributor, and her byline appears in numerous publications, including *The New York Times*, *Health Radar*, WebMD.com, CURE.com, AARP .com, GoodHousekeeping.com, and many more.

To contact Charlotte Libov:

Email: sobechar@gmail.com

Notes

_____

_____

_____

_____

_____

_____

_____

_____

_____

_____

_____

_____

_____

_____

_____

_____

_____

_____

_____

_____

Notes

Notes

Notes

Notes

Notes

Notes

You Can Live *Free* of Heart Disease

Get the tools to help you on your journey with **Crandall's Heart Health** monthly newsletter.

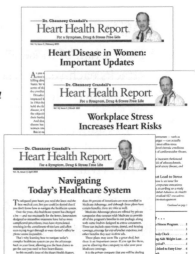

Each month *Dr. Crandall's Heart Health Report* contains effective strategies for fighting heart disease. These are the same strategies that Dr. Crandall uses with his own patients — and himself.

You'll receive information you can use immediately to help prevent and even reverse heart disease. Learn effective strategies to fight:

- **hypertension (high blood pressure)**
- **high cholesterol**
- **angina**

Plus, Dr. Crandall will share with you information on how to live:

- **symptom free**
- **drug free**
- **stress free**

This is just a fraction of the potentially life-saving information you'll receive in *Dr. Crandall's Heart Health Report*.

No matter if you've just been diagnosed with heart disease, have been battling it for years, or just want to prevent it, you'll discover every issue of *Dr. Crandall's Heart Health Report* to be an outstanding source of real-world strategies to help you live symptom free, drug free, and stress free.

Subscribe Today and Receive up to Three FREE Gifts.

CrandallReport.com/Gifts

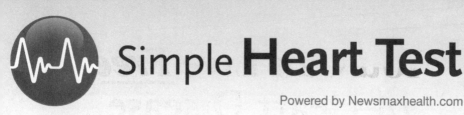

Simple **Heart Test**

Powered by Newsmaxhealth.com

FACT:

▶ Nearly half of those who die from heart attacks each year never showed prior symptoms of heart disease.

▶ If you suffer cardiac arrest outside of a hospital, you have just a 7% chance of survival.

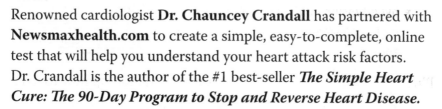

Don't be caught off guard. Know your risk now.

TAKE THE TEST NOW ...

Renowned cardiologist **Dr. Chauncey Crandall** has partnered with **Newsmaxhealth.com** to create a simple, easy-to-complete, online test that will help you understand your heart attack risk factors. Dr. Crandall is the author of the #1 best-seller *The Simple Heart Cure: The 90-Day Program to Stop and Reverse Heart Disease.*

Take Dr. Crandall's Simple Heart Test — it takes just 2 minutes or less to complete — it could save your life!

Discover your risk now.

- **Where you score on our unique heart disease risk scale**
- Which of your lifestyle habits really protect your heart
- **The true role your height and weight play in heart attack risk**
- Little-known conditions that impact heart health
- **Plus much more!**

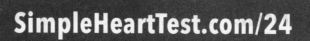

SimpleHeartTest.com/24